Vibrational Raindrop Technique

by

Christi Bonds-Garrett, M.A., M.D.

Foreword by
David Stewart, Ph.D., D.N.M.

Dedicated to my beloved husband,
Scott Garrett,
my best friend and companion
in this world
and all the worlds that follow.

Acknowledgements

Many thanks to:

Paul Horn, for my first introduction to sound healing and its amazing effects on the spirit of sentient beings, as seen in the whales he serenaded in British Columbia.

Jonathan Goldman, one of the foremost Sound Healers on the planet. In the last decade, I have continually derived inspiration from the multitude of his works, ranging from books explaining theory of sound healing to numerous CDs from which to experience firsthand healing with vibration. He emphasizes the importance of toning from within (chanting) to heal the organs, as well as the role of Intention combined with sound Frequency to create healing in his core concept of Frequency + Intention = Healing.

John Beaulieu, wayfarer on the path of Sound Healing since the 1970s, for his clarification of the importance of musical intervals as they affect our thoughts and feelings.

Hans Cousto for calculating the planetary frequencies from Keppler's work in the first place, and making this information widely known to further the healing efforts and research of individual healers all over the planet.

Donna Carey, Marjorie Mynck and Ellen Franklin for their groundbreaking work in creating Acutonics, a cohesive system in which to apply tuning forks to the Extraordinary Vessels of Chinese medicine, the storehouse of our life force. Teaming with MichelAngelo, gifted astrologer and musician, in creating detailed discussions of these vibrational intervals and their effects based upon the involved planetary body. And Jude and Paul Ponton, seasoned health practitioners, for using the forks, chimes and gongs in their busy private teaching practice to refine and clarify their uses in healing.

Dr. Andrew Weil, visionary physician who embodies the best of what one's doctor should be like: approachable, warm, wise, and with a wonderful sense of humor. And thanks to all my mentors at the University of Arizona Fellowship in Integrative Medicine program (Victoria Maizes, Randy Horowitz, Tieraona Low Dog), for continually raising the bar of excellence in delivering "the best medicine" from whatever source it comes.

Jeffrey Yuen, 88th generation Taoist priest, from whom I learned much about the use of essential oils in the context of Chinese medicine energetics. His gentle nature and personification of "cultivating the healer within" have left a strong imprint on my practice of medicine. Whenever Jeffrey came to the West Coast to lecture on essential oils, I was certain to be in the audience.

Gary Young, a true Visionary of our age, for leading the way in the cultivation, harvesting and use of essential oils, the "Missing Link" in the medicine of today and the future. We are probably too close to the ongoing accomplishments of his life to fully appreciate their enormity. Raindrop Technique epitomizes the inspired application and anointing of aromatic frequencies to the body in our quest for returning to our original state of perfection as created by the Creator.

David and Lee Stewart, who tenaciously crafted the program for CARE (Center for Aromatherapy Research and Education), making the study of the chemistry of essential oils truly simple and a joy to pursue, as well as bringing Raindrop Technique alive for me and a springboard from which to personalize and enhance its application in my professional practice as a physician.

Charles Wildbank, master visionary artist, for the exquisite cover art showing the beauty contained in the rainbow spectrum of a Raindrop.

As I contemplate the great minds and spirits of those persons mentioned herein, as well as the amazing times in which we live, I am very nearly overwhelmed at the beauty and precision of our Universe, and so much of it yet to be "discovered." I can think of no greater past-time than this: to seek out evidence of the Divine Plan in every molecule around us.

Foreword

Raindrop Technique originated in the 1980s through the research and practice of D. Gary Young. During its more than twenty-year history, it has undergone many refinements, changes, and variations.

Many of these modifications came as a consequence of the thousands taught by Gary Young over the years who added their own variations according to the perceived needs of their clients in their home areas. As a result, today there are literally hundreds of versions of Raindrop Technique seen, taught, and practiced around the world.

Many of the different versions of Raindrop that exist today actually originated from Gary Young, himself, who customarily demonstrates different ways of doing Raindrop with every seminar he teaches. His stated reason for changing things with each demonstration is to customize and adapt the procedure according to the needs of the client upon whom he is working at the time.

However, the core of the Raindrop Technique has remained relatively constant throughout the years in that the same suite of seven single oils and two blends are almost always used. Thus, the blends of Valor and AromaSeiz are always used, as well as the seven single species, namely, Oregano, Thyme, Wintergreen (or Birch), Basil, Marjoram, Cypress, and Peppermint.

In addition, the means of applying the oils in Raindrop has also remained almost the same since the beginning, consisting of Vitaflex and other simple techniques of applying fingers and hands to the feet and back.

Now Dr. Christi Bonds-Garrett has taken Raindrop Technique to another level. She hasn't changed the basic way of doing Raindrop. She consistently practices the version of Raindrop taught by D. Gary Young at a Young Living Training Workshop in Dallas, Texas, in January 2000.

There were more than 1000 participants who came from all over the world to learn Raindrop from Gary at that Seminar. Gary demonstrated Raindrop twice on two people in succession, with cameras rolling, indicating that this was to be his best and final version and that it would be published by Young Living as a VHS Video. (However, that Raindrop Video was never produced and Gary never taught it exactly like that again at any Young Living Training.)

Many, who have learned and done more than one version of Raindrop, themselves, and who have also practiced the version taught in Dallas in 2000, have concluded from their experiences that the way Gary taught Raindrop in that Dallas Seminar is one of his most effective versions. The Center for Aromatherapy Research and Education (CARE) has also come to that conclusion and has preserved Gary's original "Dallas" version of Raindrop since its founding in 2001. CARE Instructors continue to teach Raindrop that way to this day.

The version of Raindrop upon which this book is based is the one Gary taught in Dallas in 2000. It is also the one taught by CARE. It is referred to here as the "Classical Raindrop." The additional oils, outside of the nine oils of the original Raindrop, are also Gary Young's ideas. These are given on p. 299 of the 4th edition of the *Essential Oils Desk Reference* (EODR). However, these oils are only listed there, while their sequence and manner of use are not given. It was Dr. Bonds-Garrett who researched their various chemistries and vibrational characteristics to create the protocols for their applications, as presented in this book.

Dr. Bonds-Garrett is a medical doctor with certifications, internships, and residencies in psychiatry and family practice. She has also been a licensed homeopathic physician and is a student and practitioner of Chinese herbal medicine and reflexology. In addition, she is a Certified CARE Instructor and well experienced with the applications of essential oils in her years of clinical practice.

No one could be more qualified to develop Raindrop and bring it to new levels than Dr. Christi Bonds-Garrett. What you have in this book is a gift of ten types of Raindrop Technique, all based on the Classical Version, that address specific systems of the body. These ten Raindrop protocols, originated and researched by Christi, use different assortments of oils for each application. These protocols also employ the frequencies and vibrations of tuning forks that resonate with your body's systems and stimulate their healing and balance.

Through this book you now have a way to apply healing vibrations from two sources: 1. From the intrinsically high frequencies of essential oils; and 2. From actual vibrations of physical sound through tuning forks. Combining the two modalities, Dr. Bonds-Garrett has discovered and developed a set of powerful and new therapeutic protocols to address every body system in specific, targeted terms. Thus, the name "Vibrational Raindrop Technique."

In this book, Dr. Bonds-Garrett provides you with ten different Vibrational Raindrop Protocols. Starting with the Classical Raindrop, fortified by tuning forks, she presents and explains Vibrational Raindrop Techniques for Brain, Colon & Digestion, Heart & Circulation, Hormone Balance for Women, Hormone Balance for Men, Joints & Bones, Liver, Lungs, and Longevity. Whatever your needs, Christi has exactly the Raindrop that would be best for you.

All we can say is, Thank You, Doctor. This work has been a labor of love on your part and now that love is going out to bless the world through this book.

David Stewart, Ph.D., D.N.M.
Marble Hill, Missouri, USA

Table of Contents

Table of Contents cont'd

Introduction

As I sit here on a winter's day looking out over snow-covered fields from my view high above in the top floor of our Bird Wing, melodic strains of Jonathan Goldman's Celestial Reiki II fill the air, waxing and waning in volume and intensity. My usually ebullient and frisky parrots are seemingly mesmerized by this music, eyes closed shut and heads wanting to tuck under their wings. It is still morning, and this is their time of usual greatest activity. But obviously the calming effect of Jonathan's music is more powerful than the time of day.

In one way or another, I have been involved with sound and essential oils for more than 20 years. I suppose I first noticed the amazing effects of sound frequencies on animals while I was previewing Andrew Weil and Kimba Arem's CD called Self-Healing with Sound and Music. Working at the computer on another project with a deadline, I had slipped the CD into the computer's player, thinking I would accomplish two projects at the same time. Apollo, my African Grey parrot, was climbing all over my lap, trying to chew the computer keyboard, and generally making a pest of himself. The moment the first notes of Track One were played, Apollo went into a trance state: he became absolutely still, cocked his head to the side, and appeared to be lost in his thoughts as he listened to the music of didgeridoos and singing bowls. This particular CD is composed of music and sounds that move from a higher frequency of Beta brainwave activity through Alpha and Theta down to Delta, and has been used successfully for insomnia by many of my patients.

At the time, I was beginning a two-year Fellowship in Integrative Medicine at the University of Arizona under the guidance of Dr. Andrew Weil, the Harvard-trained physician whose face on book and magazine covers is a familiar site to most Americans. Indeed, Time Magazine named him one of the 25 most influential Americans in 1997 and one of the 100 most influential people in the world in 2005. Always at the forefront of integrating the best and most diverse medicine out there, Dr. Weil has created a program at the University of Arizona to educate western trained physicians in the rapidly growing field known as Integrative Medicine (IM). His Arizona Center for Integrative Medicine defines IM as "healing-oriented medicine that takes account of the whole person (body, mind, and spirit), including all aspects of lifestyle. It emphasizes the therapeutic relationship and makes use of all appropriate therapies, both conventional and alternative."

There is a lot of information packed into that definition, which describes a fundamental shift in how we practitioners of "western medicine" should deliver healthcare. It acknowledges the necessary partnership between patient and practitioner in healing-oriented medical care, and is predicated on a foundation that includes all the many factors influencing our states of health such as mind, body, spirit -- and community.

As I sit here in the Bird Wing today listening to Celestial Reiki II, I am also reminded of the flute music of Paul Horn, which I first heard in the early 1970s. In 1968 Paul, a jazz musician and musical pioneer, was in India filming a documentary. One dark night, he took his flute into the dome of the Taj Mahal and played to the stars, haunting melodies of exquisite joy. Over the years, I listened to his music frequently, and it never failed to transport me to a place of inspiration and healing.

A few years later I heard that Paul would be appearing in a small theater in Portland, Oregon. I made certain to be there. Rather than performing his Taj Mahal music, however, he presented a show about playing the flute to killer whales in British Columbia! The whales came to him at poolside, intently listening with their faces poking out of the water, leaning on the rim of the pool, nuzzling him and his flute, and eventually answering his music with their own. Most of us left the little theater that magical evening shaking our heads in wonderment, little appreciating the larger healing message that Paul was revealing to us.

The importance of sound, vibration, frequency, intention, shape/form and their interrelatedness become more obvious on a daily basis. Jonathan Goldman, a respected sound healer for decades, is well-known for his equation, "frequency + intention = healing." Throughout this book I will refer to this equation, substituting my own preferred methods of creating frequency and intention to obtain the desired outcome of healing.

Dr. Weil teaches, "Good medicine is based in good science. It is inquiry-driven and open to new paradigms." We will explore the rapidly emerging paradigm of frequency-based medicine, whether that frequency comes from the sound of tuning forks, the substance of essential oils, or other modalities which are composed of frequencies. Which, when you think about it, is just about everything!

What is Raindrop Technique?

Raindrop Technique is a method of applying therapeutic grade essential oils to the feet and back/spine using special techniques such as Vitaflex, feathered finger stroking, and dropping the oils in "raindrop" fashion onto the back. It was developed by Gary Young during the 1980s based on his knowledge of essential oils' antimicrobial effects coupled with the ability of Vitaflex and effleurage to generate electrical energy in the body.

Gary learned about the Lakota tradition of migrating north from South Dakota into Canada's northern regions to witness the Northern Lights, or Aurora Borealis. According to a Native elder, the sick among them would hold their hands to the Lights, inhaling deeply and "breathing in" this healing energy, spreading it to their spines and along neurological pathways, with subsequent dramatic healing results for many.

But when the US/Canadian border was closed and migration became impossible, the Lakota began mentally practicing this form of energy healing and substituted effleurage (feathered finger stroking) for the Northern Lights to diffuse the energy throughout their bodies.

Gary coupled effleurage with Vitaflex, which means "vitality through the reflexes." Thought to originate in Tibet, the technique was perfected in the 1960s by Stanley Burroughs and is described in detail in his book Healing for the Age of Enlightenment. Electrical energy is induced with the pressure of the pad of the fingers on the skin, and released along nerve pathways when the electrical circuit is broken as the finger tips roll over onto the fingernail.

In Raindrop Technique, essential oils are applied with Vitaflex onto reflex points primarily on the soles of the feet, though there are hundreds of Vitaflex points all over the body. Thumb Vitaflex technique is also applied along the spine. Raindrop follows the French model for aromatherapy, using undiluted essential oils. Some of the more well-known practitioners of the French model in the last 40 years include Rene Gattefosse, PhD, Jean Valnet, MD, Jean-Claude Lapraz, MD, Kurt Schnaubelt, PhD, and Daniel Penoel, MD.

For an excellent overview of Raindrop Technique's effects, *A Statistical Validation of Raindrop Technique* is essential reading. In 2001, David Stewart, PhD, tabulated 422 responses to a questionnaire about the effects of Raindrop. These questionnaires summarized the experiences of over 14,000 sessions of Raindrop. Significantly, 99.9% of persons receiving Raindrop said they would choose to receive it again. The receivers rated it positive (97%), pleasant (98%), resulted in improved health (89%) and in improved emotional state (86%).

NOTE: This book is not an instructional book about how to perform Raindrop, but rather is a guide to the use of tuning forks (sound and vibration) to augment the effects of Raindrop. For more information on performing Raindrop, please see the Bibliography and Resources sections. For a calendar of Raindrop Training Seminars visit www.RaindropTraining.com.

About Essential Oils

Essential Oils are the life blood of a plant, and are vital to the life of the plant. Most of the time they are produced by steam distillation. They are composed of hundreds of compounds that are individually very tiny, usually much smaller than 300 atomic mass units (amu, or dalton). It is because of this small size that the molecules of essential oils are aromatic; they can diffuse in the air and stimulate our sense of smell through Cranial Nerve 1.

Any single essential oil may have hundreds of different molecules. Orange oil (citrus sinensis) contains 34 alcohols, 30 esters, 20 aldehydes, 14 ketones, 10 carboxylic acids, and 36 varieties of terpenes including mono-, sesqui-, di- and tetraterpenes! Since no essential oil has been completely analyzed, this analysis of orange oil cannot be considered complete.

Essential oils perform many functions in plants as well as in people: they assist metabolism, act as types of hormones and ligands, fight off infections by viruses, bacteria, parasites and fungi, and always work towards maintaining balance, or homeostasis, within the plant or person.

An essential oil must be distilled by therapeutic grade standards in order to extract an oil that is as close to nature as possible. Distillation must be done slowly, at low pressure, and at a relatively low temperature. The chemical profile of the primary constituents must fall within the parameters and standards of AFNOR (Association French Normalization Organization Regulation) and/or ISO (International Standards Organization). There are no therapeutic grade standards in North America yet.

Therapeutic grade essential oils are the only oils that are safe to use in a therapeutic manner. Unfortunately, over 90% of the essential oils produced today are for the perfume and food industry and would not be good choices to use in Raindrop Technique. While there are other sources of therapeutic grade essential oils, this book advises the reader to use only Young Living essential oils for Raindrop Technique.

Vegetable oils (or "fatty acids" to chemists) come from the seeds of plants, are much larger than essential oils, and subsequently do not have much aroma. They are not essential to the life of the plant but instead provide nourishment to new seedlings. They can be used to slow down the absorption into the skin of an essential oil (such as using V-6 in Raindrop), or as a carrier for more dilute blends of essential oils (such as Ortho-Ease in Raindrop).

I have included some basic information on the use of the oils according to Chinese medicine interpretation since I am always thinking in that medical model as well. Chinese medical theory has a logical, codified system for the diagnosis and treatment of disease. Blood, Qi, and Yin/Yang are at the foundation of this system with Yin and Yang manifesting pathologically in concepts of cold and hot, deficiency and excess, damp and dry. They generally relate to two opposites that need to be held in balance. "Qi" is simply translated as "life force", or as "energy". Essential oils address three distinct constitutional levels described by Chinese medicine: the wei (protective meridians), ying (the 12 regular meridians and divergent meridians) and yuan (eight curious meridians, or extraordinary vessels).

Traditional Chinese Medicine (TCM) encompasses a comprehensive medical theory as well as an extensive pharmacopoeia which is organized into 24 categories by action. Each herb is explained through its energetics as well as its actions and the particular organ meridian it affects. According to Chinese herbal energetics, some herbs have ascending actions, while others descend; some invigorate while others sedate. Some herbs move to the body's surface or the extremities, while others penetrate deeply to affect organ functioning. At the root of it all is the most fundamental Kidney Qi: that which provides us with vitality and ensures proper function of all other organs.

For an absorbing look into the world of essential oils, the reader is strongly recommended to get a copy of David Stewart's *The Chemistry of Essential Oils Made Simple*. You will surprise yourself at what fascinating reading chemistry can be!

Sound, Frequency and Form

Sound is the primary creative force in the universe! Sound came first, with all of creation following. Many cultures concur with this thought:

In the book of *Genesis* from the *Old Testament*, one of the first statements is, "And God said, 'Let there be light; and there was light." God speaks the name "Light" and through this creates light. Sound came before Light. "And the Spirit of God moved upon the face of the waters" before God spoke light into being.

In the *Gospel according to John* in the *New Testament*, it is written, "In the beginning was the Word, and the Word was with God, and the Word was God." Words come from sound, and the word/sound was in the beginning. Light again comes after sound: "In him was life; and the life was the light of men."

According to Jonathan Goldman, the ancient Egyptians believed that their god Thoth would speak the name of an object, and it would come into Being. In the Vedas, it says, "In the beginning was Brahman with whom was the Word." Spider Woman of the Hopi legends sang the song of creation over the inanimate forms on earth, bringing them to life. In the Popul Vuh in Mayan tradition, the first people are given life by the power of the voice. Similar legends exist in the Australian Aboriginal traditions, Polynesia and the Far East, as well as many African tribes. They all agree that the origin of the world came through Sound.

Sound is energy in wave form which is measured in cycles per second, its frequency. Everything is in a state of vibration, and therefore everything is sound. As the ancient Sanskrit saying goes, "Nada Brahma", or "the world is sound." Sound is synonymous with God, so "the world is sound, and sound is Brahma/God." To Joachim Berendt, this means that the world vibrates in harmonic proportions, which he discusses at great length in his book The World is Sound: Nada Brahma.

In quantum physics terms, "everything is sound" relates to electrons moving around the nucleus of an atom, and planets moving around the star of their galaxy, while galaxies move around a larger Source.

We hear sound in the range from 20 to 20,000 cps, or Hertz (named after the German physicist who first discovered radio waves, Heinrich Rudolph Hertz, 1857-1894). We can also "feel" very low frequencies even when we can barely hear them. Our range of hearing diminishes as we age, with a higher range of hearing in our youth. Mice have an extremely high range of hearing and can hear sound waves up to 100,000 cps, while dolphins have a range up to 180,000 cps! Even though we cannot hear that range of frequencies, it still exists, and other animals are able to hear it and sound it. The faster the frequency, the higher (treble) the sound, and the slower the frequency, the lower (bass) the sound.

Sound creates form. One of the most well-known scientists to explore this idea was Dr. Hans Jenny, who put different substances (such as lycopodium powder) on a plate and vibrated the plate with varying frequencies of sound. The inert substance would spring to life into symmetrical shapes and designs. He also discovered that each organ of the body makes sound at specific frequencies. While they cannot be heard by the human ear, these sonic vibrations are measureable. He and a colleague in England, Dr. Peter Manners, calculated what these frequencies are. If diseased, an organ ceased emitting its key note. But when its key note was aimed at it, the diseased organ was restored to health: the diseased organs were brought back to health through resonance with a healthy frequency. Dr. Jenny's work is documented in his book *Cymatics*, and DVDs showing the shifts in patterns are available as well.

Other scientists have explored the effects of sounds on matter, and have found that specific sounds used in meditation create specific shapes. One of the most amazing examples occurred when a Buddhist monk sounded "Om" into a tonoscope, and the mandala associated with Om was created by the tonoscope! This mandala consists of multiple overlapping triangles pointing up and down, just like the symbol associated with the 6th chakra, or energy center. Sound and form are interrelated. According to Steven Halpern, "Sound is a carrier wave of consciousness."

While filming *Journey Inside Tibet* in its highlands, Paul Horn paused for a moment in the vast empty terrain and said, "you hear that stillness?... It's silence... but it's filled with potential." Like breathing with its phases of exhalation and inhalation, as well as communing with the Divine via the two phases of prayer and meditation, Sound healing has phases of audible sound and echo, or silence. This is the Still Point, from which all potential arises.

If you look at the close-up films of Dr. Jenny's tonometer while it makes geometric shapes, you will notice that the grains of powder are always moving toward the place of zero movement, or the node. The node attracts the particles of powder, which keeps the overall pattern congruent and orderly. As the tone/vibration into the tonometer is changed, the powder pauses in a still point, recognizes the new tone, and moves into the new form/pattern. As it changes form, there is a period of disorder, or chaos. The old form must break down in order for the new form to take shape.

Belgian scientist Ilya Prigogine described this phenomenon of order from chaos with his *Theory of Dissipative Structures* for which he was awarded the Nobel prize in 1977. It is in the nature of living biological systems to dissipate energy and move towards internal dissonance over time. As we move further from equilibrium/balance, a point is reached where the internal "wobble" is so great that the system breaks down into chaos, or disease. This wobble and eventual chaos is a signal that something is changing inside, or is trying to change. We need to shift into "neutral" or a Still Point, in order to facilitate the change. The more we resist, the more difficult it is to make the change with grace. Overt chaos, or disease, is frequently the result.

Let's revisit the *Old Testament*. In *Genesis*, Chapter One, it says, " In the beginning God created the heaven and the earth. And the earth was without form, and void; and darkness was upon the face of the deep." Here was the moment of chaos with the potential for a shift into a greater reality. "And God said, Let there be light and there was light." God spoke/sounded/vibrated His creation into being. Before every act of creation, at least seven more times, we find that God spoke things into being: "And God said..."

How do we assist this Still Point within us to be found? It is certainly there; God has placed it there. It is a matter of frequency tuning, and this can be done with tuning forks as well as sound or other vibrational tools, such as essential oils. Every object has a natural resonance, which is the specific frequency at which it vibrates. For optimal function, objects need to be within their natural vibration, but sometimes they shift out into an unnatural resonance. We can assist the object to find its natural and perfect resonance by entraining it with tuning fork vibrations as well as coupling it with the intention inherent in essential oils. The ability of essential oils to go deep within the body, virtually any- and everywhere, is a method to take the vibrational frequency within.

Essential Oils and Intention

Every essential oil is composed of a variety of molecular components, and each of these components has a frequency associated with it. The larger the molecule is, the more complex and the greater the spectrum of frequencies.

These frequencies are usually measured in mega-megahertz and higher. A megahertz (Mhz) vibrates at a rate of one million times per second (106 hz), and a mega-megahertz (MMhz) vibrates at a trillion times per second (1012)! Double bonds between carbon atoms vibrate between 49-68 MMhz, double bonds between carbon and oxygen atoms between 51-53 MMhz, and single bonds between carbon and oxygen between 30-39 MMhz. Conclusion: There is a lot of potential energy "zipped" into molecules of essential oils!

How do we tap into this incredible source of energy? The body has a natural intelligence and ability to access these vibrational qualities of essential oils, much like playing the keys on a piano which sets vibrating strings in motion. In modern "String Theory" the entire universe is conceived as being composed of tones like a vibrating violin string, and a pluck of a string at one point will affect all the other strings in various degrees.

A little explanation is needed here before we talk about the "useable" frequency of a molecule of essential oil. When we hear the note of C in the Pythagorean scale, we are hearing 256hz. Depending on what instrument played that note, it will sound a little different, and the identity of the instrument will be readily known. This is because of "harmonics" - the additional tones/pitches that are sent out when an instrument plays a note. These are the "color" of sound, technically known as timbre.

If two slightly different frequencies are played simultaneously, they can reinforce one another and more importantly, they can cancel out each other, leaving a smaller and more manageable frequency. What is left is the difference in frequency between the two notes. For instance, two frequencies such as 256hz and 260hz could be played, and produce a frequency as low as 10hz or less. This is called a "beat frequency." In terms of essential oils with many molecules in the mega-megaherz range, they can combine within the single oil to create a net beat frequency in the lower megaherz range. These lower beat frequencies act as the Fundamental in a harmonic group.

It is critical to note that these healing properties of essential oils apply only to pure, therapeutic grade oils! Their molecules form a coherent and harmonious family designed to heal us. If the oil is modified in any way (removing some constituents, adding synthetic ingredients, or adulterating it in other ways), it no longer is able to work in a coherent, functional way. It is like having a perfectly trained orchestra in the middle of a symphony, and a critical musician/instrument is replaced by a stranger who happens to be walking down the street. The entire orchestra will be disrupted and fall apart into dissonance.

Essential oils can also be affected by our thoughts. As described in the Higleys' Reference Guide to Essential Oils, Bruce Tainio in Washington was able to measure frequencies of people in various states of health as well as food, herbs and therapeutic grade essential oils. The healthy human ranges from 62-68Mhz overall, fresh produce 10-15Mhz, dry herbs 12-22Mhz, processed/canned foods 0Mhz, and therapeutic grade essential oils 52-320Mhz. Rose has the highest frequency (320Mhz) of single essential oils. But even more interesting is the effect that one's thoughts had on the oils. When the oils were subjected to negative thoughts, their frequencies decreased by 12Mhz, and with positive thoughts they increased by 15Mhz. Oils can serve as a vehicle to amplify intention.

Many have heard of the work of Dr. Masaru Emoto, the Japanese scientist who discovered that molecules of water are affected by our thoughts, words, and feelings. Originally conducting research into the measurement of wave fluctuations in water, he discovered that water has the ability to copy information. With some perseverance he was able to develop a method to photograph water crystals as they emerge for 20-30 seconds while the temperature rises and the ice begins to melt. He experimented with the effect of music on water, as well as words written on paper and wrapped around the water container. Water which was exposed to the music of Beethoven or Mozart showed bright, symmetrical forms, and the word "love" generated a complex and exquisite molecule. Angry words as well as exposure to microwaves and cell phones generated malformed crystals. Photographs of the resulting crystal shapes should indeed give us each pause for thought. And since humans as well as the earth are composed mostly of water, the "*Messages from Water*" are profound in their applications to us.

Essential oils, like water, have frequency and can carry intention. Since water is everywhere in our bodies, so, too, can essential oils access anywhere in the body. They have an innate wisdom that knows where to go and what to do to heal the human body. They also heal the emotions and spirit.

Intervals, Energetics & Tuning Forks

Here is a brief introduction to music theory, written by a non-musician who does understand a bit of math and astrology. Good luck!

An **interval** is the distance between two notes/tones/pitches. They are harmonic if they are sounded at the same time, while they would be called melodic if sounded in succession. A **chord** similarly is a set of three or more notes that is heard simultaneously.

There are seven main pitches or tones in the Western (**diatonic**) musical scale (A through G) and these are the white keys on a piano. But there are 12 possible notes in an octave, and then it would be called a **chromatic** scale. Five of the possible notes fall between the seven main tones; these are the black keys (sharps and flats) on a piano. Each pitch/key is the same interval away from the previous pitch/key. A sharp raises the natural note, and a flat lowers the note.

A **scale** is eight successive pitches within a one-octave range. The diatonic scale is ancient. A variation from Ptolemy in the 2nd century AD was rediscovered in the late 15th century. It has become the basic scale used in western music. An **octave** is the interval between one musical pitch and another with half or double its frequency. All scales start on one note and end on that same note one octave higher. All major scales have the same sets of distances, or intervals, between the tones. All of the notes have one whole step to the next note except 3rd to 4th and 7th to 8th. From fundamental tone/tonic to the seventh note of a diatonic Major scale, "1" represents a half step and "2" represents a whole step, the intervals of a Major scale are 2,2,1,2,2,2,1. There are twelve Major scales, each originating from one of the twelve tones that divide an octave.

There are three types of Minor scales: natural, harmonic, and melodic, and there are twelve of each type of Minor scale. A natural Minor scale is just like its corresponding Major scale, except that it starts and stops on the sixth note instead of the first/tonic note. From tonic to seventh note the whole steps (2) and half steps (1) of the Natural Minor scale are sequenced as 2,1,2,2,1,2,2.

The harmonic Minor scale is almost like the natural minor except that the seventh note is raised a half step. From tonic to seventh note the half steps (1) and whole steps are in the sequence of 2,1,2,2,1,3,1, where (3) represents an augmented whole step.

The melodic Minor scale raises both the sixth and seventh notes of the natural Minor scale by a half step each, making it easier to sing. From tonic to seventh note the sequence of whole and half steps are 2,1,2,2,2,2,1. Major scales sound happy, while Minor scales sound a little sad.

An **interval** is the sound that results when two tones/pitches are sounded at the same time. It is a point that results from the meeting of the two waves of two tones. Some intervals are naturally and traditionally pleasing to us: the octave (2:1), fifths (3:2) and fourths (4:3), where the frequencies of the two notes are proportionatly 2 to 1, 3 to 2, and 4 to 3, respectively.

Thus, Middle C on the piano vibrates at 256 Hz while the note an octave below vibrates at half that rate, or 128 Hz, hence the 2:1 ratio of frequencies. Octaves, fifths, and fourths are referred to as the "perfect intervals" in music because the ratios of the two frequencies comprising these intervals are whole numbers.

These harmonic ratios were used to create architecture long ago, and the most beautiful temples in the ancient worlds of Athens, Rome and Egypt are based upon these proportions.

A proportion known as the Golden Section was extremely important to ancient architects, and architecture has been called "music frozen in time." It says that the ratio of the whole to the larger part is the same as the ratio of the larger part to the smaller part. These proportions are found in the human body, as well as plants, insects and animals. For instance, the thigh is to the calf as the arm is to the forearm, as the lower part of the body is to the upper with the navel as the dividing point. Musically, the Golden Section is found in the ratios of the Major Sixth (3:5) and the Minor Sixth (5:8).

Music is Movement

The nature of music exists in movement. It starts from a specific point, then moves through different notes or intervals to create tension, and then releases. Consonance and dissonance arise when two notes are sounded together, creating an interval which is either pleasing and relaxing (**consonant**) or unstable, energetic and full of movement (**dissonant**). These are not absolute definitions since the response to an interval is highly subjective and related to cultural background. For instance, in the past only the first three overtones of a given fundamental were considered consonant: the unison, octave, 5th and 4th. In today's world, we experience most intervals as relatively consonant and pleasing. But the 2nds, 7ths and tritones are the most dissonant and therefore full of tension. They can be used to generate a high state of energy and movement, and are critical for growth and evolution.

I wonder if you noticed that I slipped in another word in the previous paragraph without defining it? An **overtone** is any frequency higher than the fundamental tone. Together, they are called partials and create harmonics when their frequencies are whole number multiples of the fundamental. For instance, in our system the fundamental is Ohm at 136.10hz, so overtones would have

12

frequencies in whole number multiples of Ohm, such as 272.20hz, 544.40hz, 1088.80, and on and on.

While overtones theoretically progress to infinity, we will hear them only up to about 20,000hz, or maybe not even that high depending upon your range of hearing. But remember: just because we cannot hear them, doesn't mean that they don't exist and don't have an effect! We also use lower multiples of the fundamental such as the Low Ohm with a frequency of 68.05hz. It is this spectrum of tones that range from the fundamental tone up into kilohertz of cps that gives a sound its "color" or timbre, and allows it to be differentiated from other sources (instruments) of sound.

Intervals of the tuning forks represent the "frequency" in the equation "Frequency + Intention = Healing" (Jonathan Goldman). "Intention" is represented by the use of the specific essential oil. "Healing" is the desired outcome. Thus, this equation can be rewritten as "Tuning Forks + Essential Oils = Desired Outcome."

An interval's quality is determined by its relationship to the Fundamental tone within the system being used. Two of the most common systems of tuning forks on the market today are those relating to a Fundamental of a multiple of 8 Hz (the Pythagorean scale), and those relating to a Fundamental of 136.10, which is the sound of Ohm (the sound of an Earth year, or the time it takes Earth to travel through the four seasons around the sun). In this system to enhance Raindrop, I am using the planetary tuning forks according to Cousto's calculations with the tuning fork of Ohm/136.10 as the fundamental. Together with the planetary tuning forks, the combinations create intervals with certain characteristics, as explored by Donna Cary and her colleagues at Acutonics.

Tuning Fork Intervals and Planetary Energetics

Here are some of the possible intervals that can be used with their associated musical and planetary energetics. The name of the interval is in large typeface (Unison), then its ratio (1:1), then the name of the tuning fork to be used with Ohm.

Unison, 1:1
Ohm/Ohm - centering, rooting and grounding

Microtone - interval that is less than an equally spaced semitone, which in this case would be equal to 36.66 Hz in a twelve incremental Octave. The primary microtones in this system occur near the Unison, and are necessary to assist one to move away from grounding and center, to move away from a comfort zone in order to explore new possibilities and stimulate expansion and growth from within.

Pluto/Ohm - highly dissonant, penetrates deep into the body structure to a cellular level, breaks down resistance to change, unconscious and shadow self level. Disharmony between notes creates desire for resolution.

Mercury/Ohm - creates a great deal of movement and dissonance; volatile, going between the cracks.

Minor Second, 15:16

Mars/Ohm - harsh; carrier of considerable energetic potential, propels the mind, body and spirit into action with power and initiative to remove obstacles.

Saturn/Ohm - semitone and somewhat dissonant, supports the formation of new boundaries and structures. The Minor Second is the most dissonant of the intervals, and Saturn/Ohm is more dissonant than Mars/Ohm. They both represent the applications of energy toward the manifestation of material form, in other words creating matter from spirit. Twin pillars of evolution on the material and spiritual planes.

Major Third, 4:5

Zodiac Earth/Ohm - optimistic, happy; meditative, dispersive or dispelling effect, relieves mental stress, but is especially useful to relieve physical stress.

Fourth, 3:4

Jupiter/Ohm - Perfect Fourth; pure, like church bells; stimulates growth, abundance and expansion. The Fourth is the geometric mean of an Octave.

Fifth, 2:3

The Fifth is the halfway point (harmonic mean) between octaves. A point of release from a particular paradigm. In the key of "C", this would be the notes C and G sounded together. In the key of Ohm, this would be Ohm and a frequency about 204.15hz sounded together. Many planets create a variation of the "perfect 5th", and each has its own keynote which related to the planet involved. The 5th interval is pure, like church bells (like the Perfect 4th).

The 5th interval is associated with the nitrogen atom (Berendt) and stimulates nitric oxide release by an unknown mechanism (Beaulieu 2003). Beaulieu postulates that nitric oxide acts locally as a hormone as well as a neurotransmitter, is antibacterial and antiviral, enhances the immune system, balances the heart, pituitary gland and sphenoid bone, balances the autonomic nervous system, releases opiate and cannabinoid receptor sites in the brain's third ventricle. It enhances the mobility of joints, and can relieve depression.

This interval is the foundation of Gregorian chant in which the first section sings the fundamental tone and the other section sings the Fifth Interval. Because of the resonance of European cathedrals, only one melody needs to be sung as it bounces back the harmony of the Fifth (known as the Hildegard Thumbprint after Hildegard von Bingen the 12th century mystic, herbalist and musician).

14

Earth Day/Ohm - full of movement, intense propelling energy, joyful, the Energetic Fifth. Also considered to be an Augmented 4th or Diminished 5th. Three degrees above the tritone (physical midpoint of the octave) of 191.39. This interval has also been called Crux Ansata, a transition point where spirit is redeemed from matter.

New Moon/Ohm - calming, relaxing, opening, the Serene Fifth. The New Moon 5th is dispersive for emotional issues, while the Earth Day 5th is better suited to gather and strengthen energy.

Uranus/Ohm - a Perfect Fifth, could be called the Transformative Fifth; opens with the electrical charge of transformation, can shatter pre-existing conceptions and embodies the energy of freedom and independence.

Neptune/Ohm - a near Perfect Fifth, aptly called the Ecstatic Fifth, opens and moves the visionary from transpersonal to transcendental, fulfills the yearning for connection with the Infinite.

Major Sixth, 3:5

Full Moon/Ohm - optimistic, less emotional than the Major 3rd; builds energy, brings a feeling of fullness, unveiling, and purification; the ultimate expression of Yin. Can bring a sense of magic and fulfillment; is rhythmic with a pull towards healing that allows one's potential to manifest. Known as the Golden Section, Divine Proportion, or Golden Mean.

Minor Sixth, 5:8

Venus/Ohm - a mellow sense of longing; tonifies, nourishes beauty, harmony and creative passion but has a quality of inconstancy, desire and yearning for completion. Inversion of the Major Third (4th harmonic of overtone series). A Major Third plus a Minor Sixth creates an Octave.

Minor Seventh, 5:9

Sun/Low Ohm - full of tensions wanting to resolve to a Major/minor 3rd; initiative, empowerment, vitalizing and warm, with unconditional love and the ultimate expression of yang. An inversion of the Major 2nd, and the two intervals create an Octave.

High Sun/Ohm - a bit harsh but more distant and less emotional than the Major 2nd (its inversion).

Octave, 1:2

Low Ohm/Ohm - Perfect Octave, dreams come true; brings feelings of comfort, completeness, and grounding. Creates a sense of unity.

High Sun/Sonic Sun - very warming and energizing, bright sunshine on a cloudy day.

Locations of Points to Apply Tuning Forks

KI 1 (Kidney 1, Gushing Spring) - on the sole at the border between the anterior and middle thirds of the foot, proximal to the second and third MTP joints; this point calms the spirit, revives consciousness and rescues Yang, and descends excess from the head.

KI 3 (Kidney 3, Great Ravine) - Midway between the most prominant point of the malleolus medialis and the Achilles' tendon; this point nourishes Kidney Yin (clears deficiency Heat), tonifies Kidney Yang, anchors the Qi and benefits the Lung, and strengthens the lumbar spine.

CV 4 (Conception Vessel 4, Origin Pass) - Midline of the abdomen, 4 finger widths below the umbilicus; this point fortifies the Original Qi and Essence, and warms and benefits the Kidneys, Spleen, Bladder, Small Intestine, and uterus.

CV 17 (Conception Vessel 17, Chest Center) - In the center of the chest, level with the 4th rib; this point unbinds the chest, opens energy, and allows for the heart beat and the lung breath to synchronize into a coherent pattern.

GV 2 (Governor Vessel 2, Low Back Shu) - at the base of the sacrum; this point benefits the lumbar region and legs, and dispels Wind Damp.

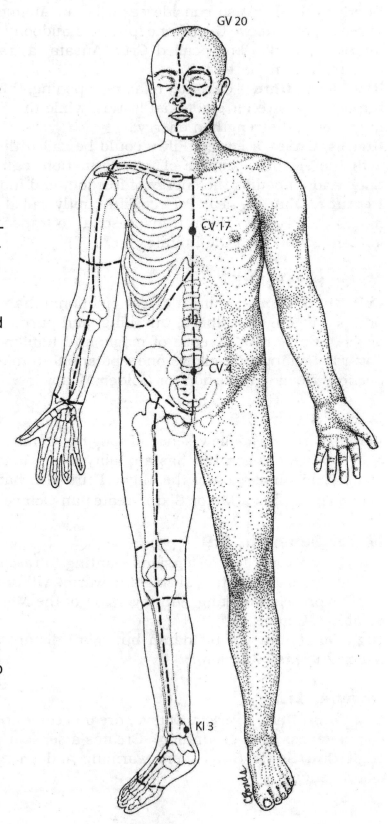

16

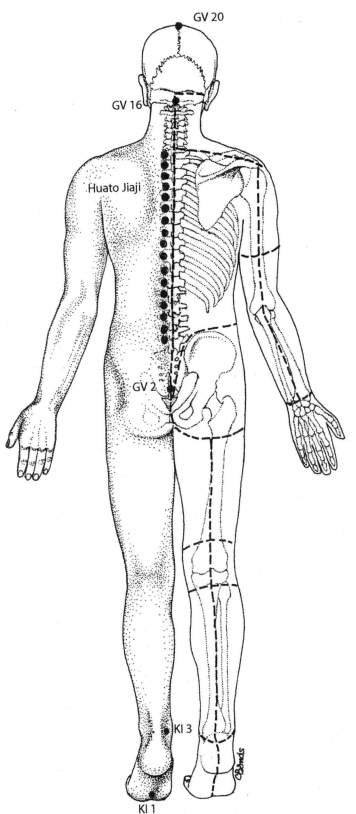

GV 16 (Governor Vessel 16, Wind Mansion) - in the depression directly below the occipital protuberance, 1 finger width above the middle of the natural hairline at the back of the head; this point calms the spirit, eliminates "wind", and benefits the head and neck.

GV 20 (Governor Vessel 20, Hundred Convergences) - on the midline of the head, about 9 finger widths directly above the posterior hairline, on the midpoint of the line connecting the apices of the ears; this point benefits the brain and calms the spirit, benefits the head and sense organs, raises Yang and counters prolapse, and nourishes the sea of marrow (brain and spinal column vitality)

Huato Jiaji - about one finger width lateral to the depressions below the spinous processes of the 12 thoracic, 5 lumbar, and 7 cervical vertebrae; these points are sounded in order to stimulate the spinal nerves.

Essential Oils & Tuning Fork Intervals
Used in Classical Raindrop Technique

Raindrop Technique is a sequence of anointing with oils and laying on of hands that brings structural and electrical alignment to the body in a relaxing and invigorating manner through the power of essential oils. There are many versions of Raindrop Technique, but the same oils are always applied, though not always in the same sequence.

Most of the Raindrop oils are high in phenolic content to ward off potentially damaging viruses and bacteria while cleansing cellular receptor sites to enhance inter- and intra- cellular communications and improve overall bodily function. Some Raindrop oils contain a variety of sesquiterpenes to assist in deleting misinformation in the DNA, as well as monoterpenes to assist in re-programming correct information into cellular memory in order to restore and maintain physical and emotional wellness.

VALOR® (contains oils of spruce, rosewood, blue tansy, and frankincense in an almond oil base) helps balance bodily electricities and stimulate spinal realignment. It affects the limbic system in a way to improve one's self-image, enhancing one's feelings of confidence, courage, and self-esteem. Contains esters, monoterpenes, and sesquiterpenes.

OREGANO (*Origanum Vulgare*) CT carvacrol - Family: Lamiaceae is one of the most powerful antimicrobial essential oils. Research at Weber State University demonstrated 99% kill rate against in vitro colonies of Streptococcus pneumoniae. High in phenolpropanoids, which cleanse cellular receptor sites.

Oregano has an affinity with the Lung, Liver, and Spleen meridians. Because oregano is warming in nature, it will warm the Middle Heater, thus strengthening Spleen qi, and expelling damp Phlegm. It can destroy parasites, and is especially useful for H. pylori.

THYME (*Thymus Vulgaris*) CT thymol - Family: Lamiaceae is antiseptic, immune enhancing, supportive of body's natural defenses. Thyme has been used to combat the bacteria that causes anthrax. High in phenolpropanoids.

With an affinity for Lung, Stomach and Kidney meridians, thyme is an excellent choice to clear Lung and Stomach Fire while tonifying Lung qi to expel phlegm. It is antiseptic and antispasmodic, and destroys intestinal worms.

BASIL (*Ocimum basilicum*) CT methyl chavicol (estragole) - Family: Lamiaceae can be relaxing to both voluntary and to the involuntary muscles as well. Voluntary muscles include all of the motor muscles of the arms, legs, back, abdomen, neck and face. Mentally energizing and invigorating . Used for tension headaches. Can improve the senses of taste and smell. High in phenolic ethers (estragole and anethole).

Basil is warming and tonifies Kidney Yang to drain Dampness in the Lower Heater; excessive use can exhaust yang energy. Especially useful for deficient Kidney Yang (infertility, low back pain, knee pain, adrenal fatigue) when applied along the Bladder/Kidney Divergent Channels along the spine. Can release Wind Cold in Yangming areas (sinuses, muscle tension, headaches), and help digest protein.

WINTERGREEN or BIRCH (*Gaultheria procumbens* or *Betula alleghaniensis*) - Family: Ericaceae (heather) or Family: Betulaceae (birch family) supports joints and skeletal structure. Composition of both of these oils are more than 80% methyl salicylate (a phenolic ester) which has a cortisone-like effect in that it may stimulate the body's own production of natural cortisone which has none of the untoward side-effects of synthetic cortisone. Also has analgesic properties inasmuch as its chemical structure is similar to that of aspirin.

Warming by nature and with an affinity for Bladder and Kidney meridians, Wintergreen expels Wind Damp Cold Bi Obstruction, so finds excellent application along the spine for chronic back problems.

MARJORAM (*Origanum marjorana*) - Family: Lamiaceae is relaxing to the involuntary muscles and to the voluntary muscles as well. Involuntary muscles include the heart, diaphragm, digestive tract, and reproductive organs. Soothing to nerves. Used for migraines. Antiseptic and antimicrobial. Marjoram is about half monoterpenes.

Marjoram has an affinity for the Lung, Liver and Stomach meridians, and is cooling in nature. It stimulates the Wei qi, and can be helpful for nervous and depressive fatigue. It descends Liver Yang qi and clears Liver Fire, so may be useful for headaches and hypertension. Marjoram expels Wind Damp Hot Bi Obstruction, and releases Wind Heat. Also promotes peristalsis and relieves reflux and flatulence by descending Stomach qi.

CYPRESS Cupressus sempervirens) - Family: Cupressaceae (cypress family) is antimicrobial. Supportive of the circulatory and lymphatic systems. Stimulates the body's natural white corpuscle production. 76% monoterpenes and 14% sesquiterpenes which may assist in restoring proper cellular programming to restore health and maintain wellness.

Slightly cooling, Cypress has an affinity for Lung, Spleen and Kidney meridians. It astringes fluid discharge that results from leakage of qi, such as urine, sweat, or diarrhea. Cypress ascends Spleen qi to upbear prolapse, hemorrhoids and varicose veins. Finally, it is very helpful to clear Lung heat and assists the Kidney to grasp Lung qi in wheezing and bedwetting.

PEPPERMINT (*Mentha piperita*) CT menthol - Family: Lamiaceae supports digestive system, respiratory system, and nervous system. Has been used for headaches. Research has shown that inhaling peppermint improves concentration and mental retention. Detoxing to the liver. A synergistic oil that supports and improves the beneficial actions of other oils used in conjunction. High in phenolics, but contains 9% sesquiterpenes.

Peppermint has an affinity for the Lung and Liver meridians with its cooling energy. Clears Wind Heat of headaches, fever, sore throat, and dry cough, as well as regulates Liver qi to promote menstruation, and decongest the Liver/PMS. It also promotes the movement of Wei qi.

AROMA SIEZ® (contains oils of basil, marjoram, lavender, peppermint, and cypress) is calming, relaxing and relieves tension. Relaxes muscles, including tight muscles and muscle spasms (seizures). May relieve headaches. Contains monoterpenes, esters and phenols.

ORTHOEASE® (a massage base oil of wheat germ, grape seed, almond, olive, and vitamin E containing essential oils of wintergreen, juniper, marjoram, red thyme, vetiver, peppermint, eucalyptus, and lemongrass) is used in European hospitals, formulated to soothe muscle aches and minor swelling. Contains natural antioxidants.

The Rainbow of Intervals Used in Classical Raindrop Technique

The ten tuning forks included in the Classic Raindrop Technique are specifically chosen to allow a full spectrum of musical intervals to be toned.

Unison - Ohm/Ohm - centering, rooting and grounding. We begin the Raindrop journey from a firm, grounded place within.

Minor 2nd - High Mars/Ohm - harsh; carrier of considerable energetic potential, propels the mind, body and spirit into action with power and initiative to remove obstacles. This interval is used near the end of the journey, when we need to mobilize our energies and courage to move and release the unnecessary burdens that we carry.

Major 3rd - Zodiac Earth/Ohm - optimistic, happy; meditative, dispersive or dispelling effect, relieves mental stress, but is especially useful to relieve physical stress. This interval is used after the Trio of oils in the middle of the Raindrop session, and it is well-suited to release muscle spasms in the back, expecially when used with Aroma Siez.

Perfect 4th - High Jupiter/High Ohm - Perfect Fourth; pure, like church bells; stimulates growth, abundance and expansion. The major energetic work of a Raindrop session has been done, and we relax for a few minutes to enjoy the bounty of it all.

Perfect 5th - Neptune/Ohm - a near Perfect Fifth, aptly called the Ecstatic Fifth, opens and moves the visionary to transcendental, fulfills the yearning for connection with the Infinite. Alternating these forks up the spine is the perfect energetic treatment for problems of the back, such as scoliosis or chronic pain.

Major 6th - High Full Moon/High Ohm - optimistic, less emotional than the Major 3rd; builds energy, brings a feeling of fullness and purification; the ultimate expression of Yin. Can bring a sense of magic and fulfillment, with a pull towards healing that allows one's potential to manifest. This interval is used as Peppermint pushes the oils ever deeper into healing levels. Relax and know that the cleansing and release are perfect.

Minor 7th - Sun/Low Ohm - full of tensions wanting to resolve to a Major/minor 3rd; initiative, empowerment, vitalizing and warm, unconditional love; the ultimate expression of Yang. This interval assists the core Duo of Oregano and Thyme to "heat up" the cells and cleanse them for deletion of old, redundant and useless information. These two points achieve "cranial-sacral stillpoint" from which changes can occur and a new order can be achieved.

Octave - Low Ohm/Ohm - Perfect Octave, dreams come true; brings feelings of comfort, completeness, and creates a sense of unity with All That Is. Thus ends our journey of healing with a Raindrop Technique session.

CLASSIC
Vibrational Raindrop

Based on Raindrop Technique as Taught by D. Gary Young
At the Young Living Level I Training Conference in
Dallas, Texas, January 25-29, 2000
(From the CARE Raindrop Training Notes)

**The notes in Underlined Helvetica Bold are the
tuning fork applications to be done with the Classic Raindrop Tuning Kit**

• **NOTE:**   The person receiving oils is called the "client" or the "receiver." The person administering the oils is called the "facilitator." While this is the version of Raindrop taught by CARE Instructors, you may adapt the tuning forks to be used after the appropriate oils in different versions of Raindrop.

• **PRELIMINARIES:** Facilitator should trim nails as short as possible and file sharp corners and edges. Facilitator and client should both remove all metal, especially rings, bracelets, and watches.

STEP 1.   EVALUATION, PREPARATION AND PERMISSION.

a.   **Measure Height** of the client barefooted using a square box against a wall and sliding down to the head to assure a level measurement. This is not an essential part of raindrop, but is an objective demonstration of what often happens. Most people grow a little with a raindrop, but if one does not grow, that does not mean the raindrop has been ineffective or erroneously per formed.

b.   **Allergies, Sensitivities, Toxicity, etc.** Ask if client is prone to allergies, reactions to drugs or has developed any sensitizations to any sub stances. Mention to the client that allergic reactions to therapeutic grade essential oils are not possible, but sometimes there can be a detox reaction. Ask if they smoke or if they have ever engaged in occu pations exposing them to chemicals such as beauty shop, auto body, professional housecleaning, pesticides, herbicides, photo chemicals, environmental engineering, hospitals, etc.

c.   **Suggested Resources with Cleansing Information**: *Essential Oils Desk Reference*; *Reference Guide for Essential Oils*; *Healing for the Age of Enlightenment*.

d.   **Ask Permission.** After explaining the procedure to the client, ask permission to continue.

e.   **Bathroom:** Ask if client needs to use bathroom before you start.

f.   **Bodily Contact:** Once session begins, the facilitator should try to keep bodily contact with client at all times. When tuning forks are sounded around the client, the facilitator will need to break bodily contact to do this technique.

- **HAVE CLIENT LIE FACE UP**

STEP 2.   VALOR®.

a.   <u>Listen to the Ohm Unison x 3 (hold tuning forks to client's ears).</u>

b.   **Shoulders.** Place 3 drops of Valor on each shoulder. Hold for 5 minutes or more until a balance of energies is felt. Place your left hand on the left shoulder and your right hand on the right shoulder.

c.   **Soles of Feet.** Place 6 drops of Valor on the soles of each foot. Cross your arms so your right hand holds the right foot and your left hand holds the left foot. You will have to cross your arms to accomplish this.

d.   <u>Sound the Ohm Unison to the sole of each foot at KI 1 (Gushing Spring) and at KI 3 (Great Ravine) in the depression behind the inner ankle x 3, right foot first.</u> We begin the Raindrop journey from a firm, grounded place within. This interval deeply roots our core essence.

STEP 3.   VALOR, OREGANO, THYME, BASIL, WINTERGREEN (or BIRCH), MARJORAM, CYPRESS and PEPPERMINT.

a.   **Foot Vita Flex.** Vita Flex on each foot along spinal reflex points, coccyx to brain, starting with right foot. Each foot should be done with 2-3 drops per foot of each of the 8 oils in the order listed x 3.

b.   <u>Sound the Ohm Octave with Low Ohm at CV4 (Origin Pass) on the abdomen four finger-widths below the umbilicus, and Ohm at CV17 (Chest Center) in the center of the chest level with the 4th rib, x 3.</u>
       This interval creates a harmonic bridge and connection between the upper and lower body, further rooting our core energy.

- **HAVE CLIENT ROLL OVER TO A FACE DOWN POSITION**

STEP 4.   DUO: OREGANO AND THYME.*

a.   **Raindrop Oregano.** Holding bottle of Oregano about six inches above the client's back, drop 4-6 drops directly on the spine from sacrum to neck.

b.   **3-6-12 Feathering Straight Up Spine.** Feather stroke Oregano straight up the spine with a light touch using backs of fingernails gently brushing against client's skin. Start with 3" strokes alternately with each hand x 3 the length of the spine upwards to the atlas vertebra, then 6" strokes x 3, followed by 12" strokes x 3.

c.   **Thyme Raindrop.** Repeat a. & b. above for Thyme.

d.   **Feathering Straight to Sides.** After both Oregano and Thyme have been applied, starting at the sacrum, feather oils away from spine straight out nd down the sides x 3, then move up half-a-hand's width and repeat until you reach the neck and skull. Repeat this sacrum to atlas x 3.

e.   **Full Length Strokes.** Long feather strokes, both hands side by side, touching with back of nail tips only along both sides of the spine, sweep full length from sacrum to base of neck, fanning out and off the shoulders x 3.

f. <u>Sound the Solar 7th with the Low Ohm on GV2 (Low Back Shu) at base of sacrum and Sun fork on GV16 (Wind Mansion) on the back of the skull one inch above the posterior hairline.</u>
This interval assists the core Duo of Oregano and Thyme to "heat up" the cells and cleanse them for deletion of old, redundant and useless information. These two points achieve "cranial-sacral stillpoint" from which changes can occur and a new order can be achieved.

*** Important Note.** *Some oils (particularly Oregano and Thyme) can cause heat when in contact with the skin and react with viruses, bacteria, and toxins. This is generally a good sign that the oils are seeking out and destroying harmful aliens that hibernate in the fatty tissue and lymph nodes along the spine. However, if at any time the heat becomes unpleasant for the client, apply V-6 or other vegetable oil where indicated. Relief should be immediate. Ask the client to tell you when and where this is needed throughout the Raindrop Technique session.*

STEP 5.   TRIO: BASIL, WINTERGREEN (or BIRCH), AND MARJORAM
a.   **Raindrop the Oils on the Back in the Order Given**. Follow steps a. & b. of STEP 4 above with Basil, Wintergreen (or Birch) and Marjoram instead of Oregano and Thyme.
b.   **Finger Circles.** After all three oils have been applied, apply your fingers to the laminar groove along one side of the spine, slowly progressing from sacrum to atlas, using four fingers of both hands together in a clockwise motion, pulling tissues away from spine with each circle. Then walk around table and go up other side. Alternate from side to side, right to left, until both sides have been done x 3. Apply Aroma Seiz® where tense muscles are discovered.
c.   <u>Sound Zodiac 3rd wherever muscle knots are found at least x 3 at each location.</u>
This interval is used after the Trio of oils in the middle of the Raindrop session, and it is well-suited to release muscle spasms in the back. If it is too painful to use the forks at the same location, then one fork can be placed on either side of the location of spasm.

Note on Additional Oils: *At this point, before the finger circles, additional oils (such as Joy®, Frankincense, Release®, Relieve It®, Harmony®, Panaway®, etc.) may be applied if desired according to the wishes, needs, or special circumstances of the client. With each additional oil, drop them raindrop-style directly on the spine and then stroke them straight up the spine with the 3-6-12 feathering described in STEPS 4a and 4b. described above.* **If other oils are added, sound the High Full Moon 6th near the client's ears, circle around head, then move in a figure eight over the client, from crown to feet and back to the crown x 3.** *Relax and know that the cleansing and release are perfect and enjoy a sense of magic and fulfillment, with a pull towards healing that allows one's potential to manifest.*

24

STEP 6.   CYPRESS.

a.   **Sprinkle Cypress.** Sprinkle Cypress oil directly on the spine with a salt-shaker-like motion from sacrum to neck.

b.   **3-6-12 Feathering Straight Up Spine**. Feather straight up spine as described in STEP 4b. x 3.

c.   **Thumb Vita Flex.** Thumb Vita Flex along sides of spine from sacrum to atlas x 3.

d.   **Saw Maneuver & Skull-Pull.** Apply saw maneuver from sacrum to neck with three skull-pulls x 3.

e.   **Spine Stretch & Shake (or Quiver).** Apply two-handed spine stretch maneuver vibrating with a shaking or quivering motion perpendicular to the spine with each stretch, moving gradually upwards from sacrum to atlas. 3x.

f.   **Sound the Neptune 5th on the Huato Jiaji points up the spine from sacrum to base of skull, alternating the Neptune and Ohm fork side to side. The Huato Jiaji points are found on either side of the spine between the vertebrae. Then hold both forks together at GV20 (Hundred Convergences) in the depression at the crown of the head and also near the ears to allow client to hear the interval.**

Alternating these forks up the spine is the perfect energetic treatment for problems of the back, such as scoliosis or chronic pain, since Neptune is associated with the spinal canal and cord.

STEP 7.   ORTHO EASE®.

a.   **Apply Ortho Ease Oil.** Dispense oil generously onto palms first, then apply over the entire back, spreading it with flat palms of the hands in clockwise circular movements from hips to neck, cross over, and then back down to the hips. Repeat x 3. A free style anointing without structure or counting may be done. Include attention of the shoulder blades, neck, trapezium muscles, and places that are tight or sore. Ask client if they have any particular requests in this regard.

b.   **(Optional) Rest.** Quietly rest face down for 4-5 minutes. Cover with sheet to keep client warm and comfortable, if necessary. Apply more Ortho Ease as needed, repeating step 7a.

c.   **Indian Rub.** Perform see-saw rub maneuver across the spine progressing from sacrum to neck and neck to sacrum, up and down the back at least x 3. Except for step 7a. above, this is the only procedure performed both up and down the back. All others are done up only, from sacrum to neck.

d.   **Sound the High Jupiter 4th near the client's ears, circle around head, then move in a figure eight over the client, from crown to feet and back to the crown x 3.**

The major energetic work of a Raindrop session has been done, and we relax for a few minutes to enjoy the bounty of it all.

CLASSIC

STEP 8.   VALOR®.

a.   Sprinkle Valor. Sprinkle Valor oil directly on the spine with salt-shaker-like motion from sacrum to neck. Valor is a mild oil blend that does not get hot and can be applied generously.

b.   3-6-12 Feathering Straight Up Spine. Feather straight up spine as described STEP 4b. x 3.

c.   Arched Feather Strokes (Angel Wings). Feather with backs of fingernails in a curved fanning motion arched up and out to sides in 3" strokes (3x), 6" strokes (3x) and 12" strokes (3x).

d.   Full Length Strokes. Long feather strokes from sacrum up to and off of the shoulders as described in STEP 4e. 3x.

e.   <u>Sound the High Mars minor 2nd near the client's ears, circle around head, then move in a figure eight over the client, from crown to feet and back to the crown x 3.</u>
We are near the end of the journey, and need to mobilize our energies and courage to expel the unnecessary burdens which we carry. Mars is associated with the adrenals and perfectly suited to resolve the imbalances associated with chronic stress.

STEP 9.   PEPPERMINT (use oil sparingly in this step, no more than 2-4 drops)

a.   Raindrop Peppermint Oil. Holding bottle of Peppermint about six inches above the client's back, drop only 2-3 drops directly on the spine from sacrum to neck.

b.   3-6-12 Feathering Straight Up Spine. Same procedure as Step 8b.

c.   Arched Feather Strokes (Angel Wings). Same procedure as Step 8c.

d.   Full Length Strokes. Same procedure as Step 8d.

STEP 10.   HOT COMPRESS.

a.   Dry Towel. Place large dry bath towel covering client's back from hips to atlas.

b.   Hot Damp Towel. Fold smaller towel into thirds, and roll into a cylinder. Then soak with hot water from the tap, wrung nearly dry, but still enough dampness to retain heat. Unroll the hot towel over the length of the spine rom neck to hips.
***Multiple Sclerosis (MS).** For people with MS, use a cold pack, NOT a hot pack. A towel soaked in cold water will do. An ice pack is also okay.

c.   Another Dry Towel. Lay another large towel over the compress to hold in heat.

d.   <u>Sound the High Full Moon Major 6th near the client's ears, circle around head, then move in a figure eight over the client, from crown to feet and back to the crown x 3.</u>
This interval is used as Peppermint pushes the oils ever deeper into healing levels. Relax and know that the cleansing and release are perfect as the Full Moon energy brings the session to fullness.

26

e. <u>**Sound the Ohm Octave to the sole of each foot at KI 1 (Gushing Spring) x 3, right foot first.**</u>
The Ohm Octave brings feelings of comfort, completeness, and creates a sense of unity with All That Is. Thus ends our journey of healing with a Raindrop Technique session.

f. **Cooking the Client.** Oils will heat up and peak out in 5-8 minutes. If heat becomes too uncomfortable, apply V-6 or vegetable oil where needed. (See Note in Step 4.) Ask client to tell you when oils have cooled to a comfortable level.

g. **If Not Hot Enough.** If oils do not heat up with client, facilitator may place hands on back over the towel. NOTE: Because peppermint oil has been applied last, the client may experience what feels like coolness when, in fact, their back is warm.

STEP 11.   REST & WATER

a. **Rest Quietly**. At this point client may wish to relax quietly for a few minutes. Whenever ready, they may sit up slowly with the facilitator standing nearby, being careful as they get off the massage table assisted by the facilitator.

b. **Drinking Water.** Have the client immediately drink a glass or bottle of good water and urge them to drink plenty of water for the next week.

STEP 12.   RE-EVALUATION AND RE-MEASUREMENT.

a. **Measure Height Afterwards**. Re-measure client's height barefooted. Most will have grown from 1/4 to 1/2 inch. Those with severe spinal curvature may grow an inch or more. The benefits of Raindrop may not always include immediate growth but can be experienced by the receiver in other ways.

b. **Adjustments Continue for a Week.** A complete evaluation of the benefits received from Raindrop Technique may take several days to assess.

c. **Drink Lots of Water.** Remind the client to drink lots of water. The recommended amount is to divide their weight in pounds by two and drink that amount in ounces of pure (non-chlorinated) water every day.

---

* These notes correspond to a 120-min DVD entitled *Raindrop Technique.*
Available from CARE, RR 4 Box 646, Marble Hill, MO 63764
• (800) 758-8629 • or visit <u>www.RaindropTraining.com</u>
Price: $29.95 • Includes a set of notes

Additional Essential Oils
Used in Raindrop Technique for Brain

All of the Systems-specific Raindrop Technique protocol use Valor, oregano and thyme as the core three oils to open and close Raindrop Technique (EDOR, 4th Ed, page 299). Basil, marjoram, wintergreen, cypress and peppermint are replaced with oils more specific to the body system being treated. Details about the specific oils used to focus on the **Brain** system are included below.

CLARITY® (contains oils of cardamom, rosemary CT cineol, peppermint, basil, bergamot, geranium, jasmine, lemon, palmarosa, Roman chamomile, rosewood and ylang ylang); promotes a clear mind and amplifies mental alertness, increases energy when tired, and brings the spirit and mind back into focus. Contains esters, oxides, transphenol (cardamom).

CARDAMOM (Elettaria cardamomum) -- Family: Zingiberaceae; antispasmodic (neuromuscular), has been used for senility, memory problems, headaches. Supports the respiratory system, good for sinus and lung infections (contains over 32% 1,8 cineole). Steam distilled from seeds which were called "Grains of Paradise" since the Middle Ages, highly prized spice in Ancient Greece and Rome. Uplifting, energizing, refreshing. High in esters (over 50%) as well as oxides (1,8 cineole). Contains high levels of transphenol, which may generate headaches in the presence of petrochemicals or heavy metals.

Warming Cardamom has an affinity for the Lung and Spleen meridians. It harmonizes Spleen and Stomach to treat digestion problems, and transforms Dampness in Summer Heat. Especially good for Rebellious Qi and Turbid Dampness with dizziness, abdominal fullness and poor concentration.

M-GRAIN® (contains marjoram, lavender, peppermint, basil, Roman chamomile, and helichrysum); has been used to relieve pain from muscular headaches as well as migraine headaches; anti-inflammatory and antispasmodic. Contains monoterpenes, phenolics, sesquiterpenes.

PEACE & CALMING® (contains blue tansy, patchouli, tangerine, orange, and ylang ylang); promotes relaxation and a deep sense of emotional well being; helps to dampen tensions and uplift spirits. Citrus fragrances have been shown to lessen depression and increase a deep sense of security (Mie University, 1995). Contains ketones, sesquiterpenes in patchouli which stimulate the limbic center of the brain, esters and aldehydes in tangerine that are sedating and calming, monoterpenes in orange to reprogram the cells back to original perfection, and sesquiterpenes and esters in ylang ylang.

PEPPERMINT (Mentha piperita) CT menthol - Family: Lamiaceae supports digestive system, respiratory system, and nervous system. Has been used for headaches. Research has shown that inhaling peppermint improves concentration and mental retention. Detoxing to the liver. A synergistic oil that supports and improves the beneficial actions of other oils used in conjunction. High in phenolics, but contains 9% sesquiterpenes.

Peppermint has an affinity for the Lung and Liver meridians with its cooling energy. Clears Wind Heat of headaches, fever, sore throat, and dry cough, as well as regulates Liver qi to promote menstruation, and decongest the Liver/PMS. It also promotes the movement of Wei qi.

A Note About Sesquiterpenes:

Sesquiterpenes, a type of terpene commonly found in essential oils, are able to pass through the blood-brain barrier to enter the brain. This barrier separates our circulating blood from the brain in order to protect the brain from exposure to toxins that the rest of the body can tolerate. However, there are certain diseases that can be treated only by access via the blood-brain barrier: Alzheimer's disease, multiple sclerosis, Parkinson's disease to name a few. Sesquiterpenes are able to carry oxygen into the cells all over the body, including the brain. Both frankincense and sandalwood have significant levels of sesquiterpenes and sesquiterpenols, which can increase the oxygenation of the limbic system in the brain. This affects the pituitary and pineal glands, critical to our bodies' functioning. It also affects the amygdala, a key player in the storage and releasing of emotional trauma. Other oils with high levels of sesquiterpenes include vetiver, vitex, cedarwood, black pepper, ylang ylang, melissa, myrrh, goldenrod, German chamomile, patchouli, ginger, spikenard, and copaiba.

Additional Intervals
Used in Brain Raindrop Technique

High Mercury/High Ohm - creates a great deal of movement and dissonance; volatile, going between the cracks, mental illumination and communication. Mercury has an affinity with the nervous system and communication of all kinds. It also balances the sympathetic nervous system and thyroid.

Uranus/Ohm - A Perfect Fifth, the Electrical Fifth; opens with the electrical charge of transformation, can shatter pre-existing conceptions and embodies the energy of freedom and independence. Mentally transformative, illuminating, inventive and break-through ideas. Uranus governs the electrical activity of the nervous system, and can calm and balance it.

BRAIN
Vibrational Raindrop

Based on Raindrop Technique as Taught by D. Gary Young
At the Young Living Level I Training Conference in
Dallas, Texas, January 25-29, 2000
(From the CARE Raindrop Training Notes)

**The notes in Underlined Helvetica Bold are the
tuning fork applications to be done with the Brain Raindrop Tuning Kit**

• **NOTE:**   The person receiving oils is called the "client" or the "receiver." The person administering the oils is called the "facilitator." While this is the version of Raindrop taught by CARE Instructors, you may adapt the tuning forks to be used after the appropriate oils in different versions of Raindrop.

• **PRELIMINARIES:** Facilitator should trim nails as short as possible and file sharp corners and edges. Facilitator and client should both remove all metal, especially rings, bracelets, and watches.

STEP 1.   EVALUATION, PREPARATION AND PERMISSION.

a.   **Measure Height** of the client barefooted using a square box against a wall and sliding down to the head to assure a level measurement. This is not an essential part of raindrop, but is an objective demonstration of what often happens. Most people grow a little with a raindrop, but if one does not grow, that does not mean the raindrop has been ineffective or erroneously per   formed.

b.   **Allergies, Sensitivities, Toxicity, etc.** Ask if client is prone to allergies, reactions to drugs or has developed any sensitizations to any sub stances. Mention to the client that allergic reactions to therapeutic grade essential oils are not possible, but sometimes there can be a detox reaction. Ask if they smoke or if they have ever engaged in occu pations exposing them to chemicals such as beauty shop, auto body, professional housecleaning, pesticides, herbicides, photo chemicals, environmental engineering, hospitals, etc.

c.   **Suggested Resources with Cleansing Information**: *Essential Oils Desk Reference*; *Reference Guide for Essential Oils*; *Healing for the Age of Enlightenment*.

d.   **Ask Permission.** After explaining the procedure to the client, ask permission to continue.

e.   **Bathroom:** Ask if client needs to use bathroom before you start.

f.   **Bodily Contact:** Once session begins, the facilitator should try to keep bodily contact with client at all times. When tuning forks are sounded around the client, the facilitator will need to break bodily contact to do this technique.

30

• HAVE CLIENT LIE FACE UP

STEP 2. VALOR®.

a. <u>**Listen to the Ohm Unison x 3 (hold tuning forks to client's ears).**</u>

b. **Shoulders.** Place 3 drops of Valor on each shoulder. Hold for 5 minutes or more until a balance of energies is felt. Place your left hand on the left shoulder and your right hand on the right shoulder.

c. **Soles of Feet.** Place 6 drops of Valor on the soles of each foot. Cross your arms so your right hand holds the right foot and your left hand holds the left foot. You will have to cross your arms to accomplish this.

d. <u>**Sound the Ohm Unison to the sole of each foot at KI 1 (Gushing Spring) and at KI 3 (Great Ravine) in the depression behind the inner ankle x 3, right foot first.**</u> We begin the Raindrop journey from a firm, grounded place within. This interval deeply roots our core essence.

STEP 3. VALOR, OREGANO, THYME, CLARITY, CARDAMOM, M-GRAIN, PEACE & CALMING and PEPPERMINT.

a. **Foot Vita Flex.** Vita Flex on each foot along spinal reflex points, coccyx to brain, starting with right foot. Each foot should be done with 2-3 drops per foot of each of the 8 oils in the order listed x 3.

b. <u>**Sound the Ohm Octave with Low Ohm at CV4 (Origin Pass) on the abdomen four finger-widths below the umbilicus, and Ohm at CV17 (Chest Center) in the center of the chest level with the 4th rib, x 3.**</u> This interval creates a harmonic bridge and connection between the upper and lower body, further rooting our core energy.

• HAVE CLIENT ROLL OVER TO A FACE DOWN POSITION

STEP 4. DUO: OREGANO AND THYME.*

a. **Raindrop Oregano.** Holding bottle of Oregano about six inches above the client's back, drop 4-6 drops directly on the spine from sacrum to neck.

b. **3-6-12 Feathering Straight Up Spine.** Feather stroke Oregano straight up the spine with a light touch using backs of fingernails gently brushing against client's skin. Start with 3" strokes alternately with each hand x 3 the length of the spine upwards to the atlas vertebra, then 6" strokes x 3, followed by 12" strokes x 3.

c. **Thyme Raindrop.** Repeat a. & b. above for Thyme.

d. **Feathering Straight to Sides.** After both Oregano and Thyme have been applied, starting at the sacrum, feather oils away from spine straight out nd down the sides x 3, then move up half-a-hand's width and repeat until you reach the neck and skull. Repeat this sacrum to atlas x 3.

e. **Full Length Strokes.** Long feather strokes, both hands side by side, touching with back of nail tips only along both sides of the spine, sweep full length from sacrum to base of neck, fanning out and off the shoulders x 3.

f. **Sound the Solar 7th with the Low Ohm on GV2 (Low Back Shu) at base of sacrum and Sun fork on GV16 (Wind Mansion) on the back of the skull one inch above the posterior hairline.**
This interval assists the core Duo of Oregano and Thyme to "heat up" the cells and cleanse them for deletion of old, redundant and useless information. These two points achieve "cranial-sacral stillpoint" from which changes can occur and a new order can be achieved.

* Important Note. Some oils (particularly Oregano and Thyme) can cause heat when in contact with the skin and react with viruses, bacteria, and toxins. This is generally a good sign that the oils are seeking out and destroying harmful aliens that hibernate in the fatty tissue and lymph nodes along the spine. However, if at any time the heat becomes unpleasant for the client, apply V-6 or other vegetable oil where indicated. Relief should be immediate. Ask the client to tell you when and where this is needed throughout the Raindrop Technique session.

STEP 5. TRIO: CLARITY, CARDAMOM, AND M-GRAIN
a. **Raindrop the Oils on the Back in the Order Given.** Follow steps a. & b. of STEP 4 above with Clarity, Cardamom, and M-Grain instead of Oregano and Thyme.
b. **Finger Circles.** After all three oils have been applied, apply your fingers to the laminar groove along one side of the spine, slowly progressing from sacrum to atlas, using four fingers of both hands together in a clockwise motion, pulling tissues away from spine with each circle. Then walk around table and go up other side. Alternate from side to side, right to left, until both sides have been done x 3. Apply AromaSiez® where tense muscles are discovered.
c. **Sound Zodiac 3rd wherever muscle knots are found at least x 3 at each location.**
If it is too painful to use the forks at the same location, then one fork can be placed on either side of the location of spasm.

*Note on Additional Oils: At this point, before the finger circles, additional oils (such as Joy®, Frankincense, Release®, Relieve It®, Harmony®, Panaway®, etc.) may be applied if desired according to the wishes, needs, or special circumstances of the client. With each additional oil, drop them raindrop-style directly on the spine and then stroke them straight up the spine with the 3-6-12 feathering described in STEPS 4a and 4b. described above. **If other oils are added, sound the High Full Moon 6th near the client's ears, circle around head, then move in a figure eight over the client, from crown to feet and back to the crown x 3.** Relax and know that the cleansing and release are perfect and enjoy a sense of magic and fulfillment, with a pull towards healing that allows one's potential to manifest.*

BRAIN

STEP 6.   PEACE & CALMING®.

a. **Sprinkle Peace & Calming.** Sprinkle Cypress oil directly on the spine with a salt-shaker-like motion from sacrum to neck.

b. **3-6-12 Feathering Straight Up Spine.** Feather straight up spine as described in STEP 4b. x 3.

c. **Thumb Vita Flex.** Thumb Vita Flex along sides of spine from sacrum to atlas x 3.

d. **Saw Maneuver & Skull-Pull.** Apply saw maneuver from sacrum to neck with three skull-pulls x 3.

e. <u>**Sound the High Mercury Microtone up/above the spine and around the head x 3.**</u>
Mercury has an affinity with the nervous system and communication of all kinds. It also balances the sympathetic nervous system and thyroid.

f. **Spine Stretch & Shake (or Quiver).** Apply two-handed spine stretch maneuver vibrating with a shaking or quivering motion perpendicular to the spine with each stretch, moving gradually upwards from sacrum to atlas. 3x.

g. <u>**Sound the Uranus 5th on the Huato Jiaji points up the spine from sacrum to base of skull and up over the crown of the head. The Huato Jiaji points are found on either side of the spine between the vertebrae. Pay special attention to the neck and skull because of its relationship to the brain.**</u>
Uranus governs the electrical activity of the nervous system, and can calm and balance it.

STEP 7.   ORTHO EASE®.

a. **Apply Ortho Ease Oil.** Dispense oil generously onto palms first, then apply over the entire back, spreading it with flat palms of the hands in clockwise circular movements from hips to neck, cross over, and then back down to the hips. Repeat x 3. A free style anointing without structure or counting may be done. Include attention of the shoulder blades, neck, trapezium muscles, and places that are tight or sore. Ask client if they have any particular requests in this regard.

b. **(Optional) Rest.** Quietly rest face down for 4-5 minutes. Cover with sheet to keep client warm and comfortable, if necessary. Apply more Ortho Ease as needed, repeating step 7a.

c. **Indian Rub.** Perform see-saw rub maneuver across the spine progressing from sacrum to neck and neck to sacrum, up and down the back at least x 3. Except for step 7a. above, this is the only procedure performed both up and down the back. All others are done up only, from sacrum to neck.

d. <u>**Sound the High Jupiter 4th near the client's ears, circle around head, then move in a figure eight over the client, from crown to feet and back to the crown x 3.**</u>
The major energetic work of a Raindrop session has been done, and we relax for a few minutes to enjoy the bounty of it all.

33

STEP 8.   VALOR®.

a. **Sprinkle Valor.** Sprinkle Valor oil directly on the spine with salt-shaker-like motion from sacrum to neck. Valor is a mild oil blend that does not get hot and can be applied generously.

b. **3-6-12 Feathering Straight Up Spine.** Feather straight up spine as described STEP 4b. x 3.

c. **Arched Feather Strokes (Angel Wings).** Feather with backs of fingernails in a curved fanning motion arched up and out to sides in 3" strokes (3x), 6" strokes (3x) and 12" strokes (3x).

d. **Full Length Strokes.** Long feather strokes from sacrum up to and off of the shoulders as described in STEP 4e. 3x.

e. <u>**Sound the High Mars minor 2nd near the client's ears, circle around head, then move in a figure eight over the client, from crown to feet and back to the crown x 3.**</u>
    We are near the end of the journey, and need to mobilize our energies and courage to expel the unnecessary burdens which we carry. Mars is associated with the adrenals and perfectly suited to resolve the imbalances associated with chronic stress.

STEP 9.   PEPPERMINT (use oil sparingly, no more than 2-4 drops)

a. **Raindrop Peppermint Oil.** Holding bottle of Peppermint about six inches above the client's back, drop only 2-3 drops directly on the spine from sacrum to neck.

b. **3-6-12 Feathering Straight Up Spine.** Same procedure as Step 8b.

c. **Arched Feather Strokes (Angel Wings).** Same procedure as Step 8c.

d. **Full Length Strokes.** Same procedure as Step 8d.

STEP 10.   HOT COMPRESS.

a. **Dry Towel.** Place a large dry bath towel covering client's back from hips to atlas.

b. **Hot Damp Towel.** Fold smaller towel into thirds, and roll into a cylinder. Then soak with hot water from the tap, wrung nearly dry, but still enough dampness to retain heat. Unroll the hot towel over the length of the spine rom neck to hips.
    * Multiple Sclerosis (MS). For people with MS, use a cold pack, NOT a hot pack. A towel soaked in cold water will do. An ice pack is also okay.

c. **Another Dry Towel.** Lay another large towel over the compress to hold in heat.

d. <u>**Sound the High Full Moon Major 6th near the client's ears, circle around head, then move in a figure eight over the client, from crown to feet and back to the crown x 3.**</u>
    This interval is used as Peppermint pushes the oils ever deeper into healing levels. Relax and know that the cleansing and release are perfect as the Full Moon energy brings the session to fullness.

e. <u>Sound the Ohm Octave to the sole of each foot at KI 1 (Gushing Spring) x 3, right foot first.</u>
The Ohm Octave brings feelings of comfort, completeness, and creates a sense of unity with All That Is. Thus ends our journey of healing with a Raindrop Technique session.

f. Cooking the Client. Oils will heat up and peak out in 5-8 minutes. If heat becomes too uncomfortable, apply V-6 or vegetable oil where needed. (See Note in Step 4.) Ask client to tell you when oils have cooled to a comfortable level.

g. If Not Hot Enough. If oils do not heat up with client, facilitator may place hands on back over the towel. NOTE: Because peppermint oil has been applied last, the client may experience what feels like coolness when, in fact, their back is warm.

STEP 11. REST & WATER
a. Rest Quietly. At this point client may wish to relax quietly for a few minutes. Whenever ready, they may sit up slowly with the facilitator standing nearby, being careful as they get off the massage table assisted by the facilitator.

b. Drinking Water. Have the client immediately drink a glass or bottle of good water and urge them to drink plenty of water for the next week.

STEP 12. RE-EVALUATION AND RE-MEASUREMENT.
a. Measure Height Afterwards. Re-measure client's height barefooted. Most will have grown from 1/4 to 1/2 inch. Those with severe spinal curvature may grow an inch or more. The benefits of Raindrop may not always include immediate growth but can be experienced by the receiver in other ways.

b. Adjustments Continue for a Week. A complete evaluation of the benefits received from Raindrop Technique may take several days to assess.

c. Drink Lots of Water. Remind the client to drink lots of water. The recommended amount is to divide their weight in pounds by two and drink that amount in ounces of pure (non-chlorinated) water every day. Additional

---

* These notes correspond to a 120-min DVD entitled *Raindrop Technique*.
Available from CARE, RR 4 Box 646, Marble Hill, MO 63764
• (800) 758-8629 • or visit www.RaindropTraining.com.
Price: $29.95 + $9 s&h • Includes a set of notes

Essential Oils Used
in Raindrop Technique for Colon/Digestion

All of the Systems-specific Raindrop Technique protocol use Valor, oregano and thyme as the core three oils to open and close Raindrop Technique (EDOR, 4th Ed, page 299). Basil, marjoram, wintergreen, cypress and peppermint are replaced with oils more specific to the body system being treated. Details about the specific oils used to focus on the **Colon/Digestion** system are included below.

DI-GIZE® (contains tarragon, ginger, peppermint, juniper, fennel, lemongrass, anise, and patchouli); relieves digestive problems including indigestion, heartburn, gas and bloating. Combats candida and parasite infestation.

TARRAGON (*Artemisia dracunculus*) -- Family: Asteraceae; antispasmodic, anti-inflammatory, antifermentation, antiparasitic, digestive aid. Used in intestinal disorders, colitis, nausea; may balance the autonomic nervous system. High in phenolic ethers (estragole) and monoterpenes.

Tarragon is warming by nature with an affinity for the Liver and Spleen meridians. It regulates Stomach qi for problems such as vomiting, hiccups, belching, flatulence, dyspepsia and poor appetite. It can also be used for the Liver Qi Stagnation of PMS to promote menstruation.

CUMIN (*Cuminum cyminum*) -- Family: Apiaceae; distilled from seeds, used for digestion and infections. Immune stimulant, liver protectant. High in monoterpenes and aldehydes.

Cumin is slightly warming with an affinity for the Liver, Spleen and Heart meridians. It is indicated for Deficient Spleen qi symptoms of poor digestion, loose stools, abdominal distention, obesity and edema. It can also be used to Invigorate the Blood with Deficient Heart qi symptoms of fatigue, palpitations and low blood pressure.

FENNEL (*Foeniculum vulgare*) -- Family: Apiaceae; may be used for indigestion, constipation, balancing hormones, and PMS. It may break up fluids and toxins to cleanse the tissues. High in phenolic ethers (anethole) and monoterpenes.

Fennel has an affinity for Liver, Spleen, Stomach and Kidney meridians, and is warming. Can be used for Cold in the Liver and Stomach Channels with symptoms of abdominal pain, constipation, and difficulty with urination or menstruation. It warms the Middle Heater to promote digestion and strengthens the Kidney and Ming Men Fire (willpower).

SPEARMINT (*Mentha spicata*) - Family: Lamiaceae; can increase metabolism, stimulate the gallbladder; has been used for digestive disorders, as well as release of emotional blocks. High in ketones (carvone).

Cooling Spearmint has an affinity for the Lung and Liver meridians and promotes Wei qi movement to relieve muscular and digestive spasms, as well as clears Wind Heat.

Additional Intervals Used In Colon/Digestion Raindrop Technique

Microtone - interval that is less than an equally spaced semitone, which in this case would be equal to 36.66 Hz in a twelve incremental Octave. The primary microtones in this system occur near the Unison, and are necessary to assist one to move away from grounding and center, to move away from a comfort zone in order to explore new possibilities and stimulate expansion and growth from within.

Pluto/Ohm - highly dissonant, penetrates deep into the body structure to a cellular level, breaks down resistance to change, unconscious and shadow self level. Pluto rules the elimination of toxic wastes from the body, and assists in all bowel disharmonies.

Fifth, 2:3

High Earth Day/High Ohm - highly energetic, full of movement, intense propelling energy, joyful. Also considered to be an Augmented 4th or Diminished 5th. This interval has also been called Crux Ansata, a transition point where spirit is redeemed from matter. This interval is the most fundamental one to build energy and eliminate fatigue. We use it near the end of the session, when one's energetic stores need to be nourished and consolidated.

COLON & DIGESTION
Vibrational Raindrop

Based on Raindrop Technique as Taught by D. Gary Young
At the Young Living Level I Training Conference in
Dallas, Texas, January 25-29, 2000
(From the CARE Raindrop Training Notes)

**The notes in Underlined Helvetica Bold are the tuning fork applications
to be done with the Colon/Digestion Raindrop Tuning Kit**

• **NOTE:** The person receiving oils is called the "client" or the "receiver." The person administering the oils is called the "facilitator." While this is the version of Raindrop taught by CARE Instructors, you may adapt the tuning forks to be used after the appropriate oils in different versions of Raindrop.

• **PRELIMINARIES:** Facilitator should trim nails as short as possible and file sharp corners and edges. Facilitator and client should both remove all metal, especially rings, bracelets, and watches.

STEP 1.   EVALUATION, PREPARATION AND PERMISSION.

a.   **Measure Height** of the client barefooted using a square box against a wall and sliding down to the head to assure a level measurement. This is not an essential part of raindrop, but is an objective demonstration of what often happens. Most people grow a little with a raindrop, but if one does not grow, that does not mean the raindrop has been ineffective or erroneously per formed.

b.   **Allergies, Sensitivities, Toxicity, etc.** Ask if client is prone to allergies, reactions to drugs or has developed any sensitizations to any sub stances. Mention to the client that allergic reactions to therapeutic grade essential oils are not possible, but sometimes there can be a detox reaction. Ask if they smoke or if they have ever engaged in occu pations exposing them to chemicals such as beauty shop, auto body, professional housecleaning, pesticides, herbicides, photo chemicals, environmental engineering, hospitals, etc.

c.   **Suggested Resources with Cleansing Information**: *Essential Oils Desk Reference*; *Reference Guide for Essential Oils*; *Healing for the Age of Enlightenment.*

d.   **Ask Permission.** After explaining the procedure to the client, ask permission to continue.

e.   **Bathroom:** Ask if client needs to use bathroom before you start.

f.   **Bodily Contact:** Once session begins, the facilitator should try to keep bodily contact with client at all times. When tuning forks are sounded around the client, the facilitator will need to break bodily contact to do this technique.

38

• HAVE CLIENT LIE FACE UP

STEP 2.   VALOR®.
a.   <u>Listen to the Ohm Unison x 3 (hold tuning forks to client's ears).</u>
b.   **Shoulders.** Place 3 drops of Valor on each shoulder. Hold for 5 minutes or more until a balance of energies is felt. Place your left hand on the left shoulder and your right hand on the right shoulder.
c.   **Soles of Feet.** Place 6 drops of Valor on the soles of each foot. Cross your arms so your right hand holds the right foot and your left hand holds the left foot. You will have to cross your arms to accomplish this.
d.   <u>Sound the Ohm Unison to the sole of each foot at KI 1 (Gushing Spring) and at KI 3 (Great Ravine) in the depression behind the inner ankle x 3, right foot first.</u> We begin the Raindrop journey from a firm, grounded place within. This interval deeply roots our core essence.

STEP 3.   VALOR, OREGANO, THYME, CUMIN, TARRAGON, DIGIZE, FENNEL and SPEARMINT.
a.   **Foot Vita Flex.** Vita Flex on each foot along spinal reflex points, coccyx to brain, starting with right foot. Each foot should be done with 2-3 drops per foot of each of the 8 oils in the order listed x 3.
b.   <u>Sound the Ohm Octave with Low Ohm at CV4 (Origin Pass) on the abdomen four finger-widths below the umbilicus, and Ohm at CV17 (Chest Center) in the center of the chest level with the 4th rib, x 3.</u> This interval creates a harmonic bridge and connection between the upper and lower body, further rooting our core energy.

• HAVE CLIENT ROLL OVER TO A FACE DOWN POSITION

STEP 4.   DUO: OREGANO AND THYME.*
a.   **Raindrop Oregano.** Holding bottle of Oregano about six inches above the client's back, drop 4-6 drops directly on the spine from sacrum to neck.
b.   **3-6-12 Feathering Straight Up Spine.** Feather stroke Oregano straight up the spine with a light touch using backs of fingernails gently brushing against client's skin. Start with 3" strokes alternately with each hand x 3 the length of the spine upwards to the atlas vertebra, then 6" strokes x 3, followed by 12" strokes x 3.
c.   **Thyme Raindrop.** Repeat a. & b. above for Thyme.
d.   **Feathering Straight to Sides.** After both Oregano and Thyme have been applied, starting at the sacrum, feather oils away from spine straight out nd down the sides x 3, then move up half-a-hand's width and repeat until you reach the neck and skull. Repeat this sacrum to atlas x 3.
e.   **Full Length Strokes.** Long feather strokes, both hands side by side, touching with back of nail tips only along both sides of the spine, sweep full length from sacrum to base of neck, fanning out and off the shoulders x 3.

f. <u>**Sound the Solar 7th with the Low Ohm on GV2 (Low Back Shu) at base of sacrum and Sun fork on GV16 (Wind Mansion) on the back of the skull one inch above the posterior hairline.**</u>

This interval assists the core Duo of Oregano and Thyme to "heat up" the cells and cleanse them for deletion of old, redundant and useless information. These two points achieve "cranial-sacral stillpoint" from which changes can occur and a new order can be achieved.

__Important Note.__ Some oils (particularly Oregano and Thyme) can cause heat when in contact with the skin and react with viruses, bacteria, and toxins. This is generally a good sign that the oils are seeking out and destroying harmful aliens that hibernate in the fatty tissue and lymph nodes along the spine. However, if at any time the heat becomes unpleasant for the client, apply V-6 or other vegetable oil where indicated. Relief should be immediate. Ask the client to tell you when and where this is needed throughout the Raindrop Technique session.

STEP 5.   TRIO: CUMIN, TARRAGON AND DIGIZE.

a. **Raindrop the Oils on the Back in the Order Given**. Follow steps a. & b. of STEP 4 above with Cumin, Tarragon and DiGize instead of Oregano and Thyme.

b. **Finger Circles.** After all three oils have been applied, apply your fingers to the laminar groove along one side of the spine, slowly progressing from sacrum to atlas, using four fingers of both hands together in a clockwise motion, pulling tissues away from spine with each circle. Then walk around table and go up other side. Alternate from side to side, right to left, until both sides have been done x 3. Apply AromaSiez® where tense muscles are discovered.

c. <u>**Sound Zodiac 3rd wherever muscle knots are found at least x 3 at each location.**</u>

If it is too painful to use the forks at the same location, then one fork can be placed on either side of the location of spasm.

__Note on Additional Oils:__ At this point, before the finger circles, additional oils (such as Joy®, Frankincense, Release®, Relieve It®, Harmony®, Panaway®, etc.) may be applied if desired according to the wishes, needs, or special circumstances of the client. With each additional oil, drop them raindrop-style directly on the spine and then stroke them straight up the spine with the 3-6-12 feathering described in STEPS 4a and 4b. described above. <u>**If other oils are added, sound the High Full Moon 6th near the client's ears, circle around head, then move in a figure eight over the client, from crown to feet and back to the crown x 3.**</u> *Relax and know that the cleansing and release are perfect and enjoy a sense of magic and fulfillment, with a pull towards healing that allows one's potential to manifest.*

STEP 6.   FENNEL.

a.   **Sprinkle Fennel.** Sprinkle Fennel oil directly on the spine with a salt-shaker-like motion from sacrum to neck.

b.   **3-6-12 Feathering Straight Up Spine.** Feather straight up spine as described in STEP 4b. x 3.

c.   **Thumb Vita Flex.** Thumb Vita Flex along sides of spine from sacrum to atlas x 3.

d.   **Saw Maneuver & Skull-Pull.** Apply saw maneuver from sacrum to neck with three skull-pulls x 3.

e.   **Spine Stretch & Shake (or Quiver).** Apply two-handed spine stretch maneuver vibrating with a shaking or quivering motion perpendicular to the spine with each stretch, moving gradually upwards from sacrum to atlas. 3x.

f.   **Sound the Pluto Microtone on the Huato Jiaji points up the spine from sacrum to base of skull and up over the crown of the head. The Huato Jiaji points are found on either side of the spine between the vertebrae. Then hold both forks together at GV20 (Hundred Convergences) in the depression at the crown of the head and also near the ears to allow client to hear the interval.**
Pluto rules the elimination of toxic wastes from the body, and assists in all bowel disharmonies.

STEP 7.   ORTHO EASE®.

a.   **Apply Ortho Ease Oil.** Dispense oil generously onto palms first, then apply over the entire back, spreading it with flat palms of the hands in clockwise circular movements from hips to neck, cross over, and then back down to the hips. Repeat x 3. A free style anointing without structure or counting may be done. Include attention of the shoulder blades, neck, trapezium muscles, and places that are tight or sore. Ask client if they have any particular requests in this regard.

b.   **(Optional) Rest.** Quietly rest face down for 4-5 minutes. Cover with sheet to keep client warm and comfortable, if necessary. Apply more Ortho Ease as needed, repeating step 7a.

c.   **Indian Rub.** Perform see-saw rub maneuver across the spine progressing from sacrum to neck and neck to sacrum, up and down the back at least x 3. Except for step 7a. above, this is the only procedure performed both up and down the back. All others are done up only, from sacrum to neck.

d.   **Sound the High Jupiter 4th near the client's ears, circle around head, then move in a figure eight over the client, from crown to feet and back to the crown x 3.**
The major energetic work of a Raindrop session has been done, and we relax for a few minutes to enjoy the bounty of it all.

STEP 8. VALOR®.

a. **Sprinkle Valor.** Sprinkle Valor oil directly on the spine with salt-shaker-like motion from sacrum to neck. Valor is a mild oil blend that does not get hot and can be applied generously.

b. **3-6-12 Feathering Straight Up Spine.** Feather straight up spine as described STEP 4b. x 3.

c. **Arched Feather Strokes (Angel Wings).** Feather with backs of fingernails in a curved fanning motion arched up and out to sides in 3" strokes (3x), 6" strokes (3x) and 12" strokes (3x).

d. **Full Length Strokes.** Long feather strokes from sacrum up to and off of the shoulders as described in STEP 4e. 3x.

e. <u>**Sound the High Earth Day 5th near the client's ears, circle around head, then move in a figure eight over the client, from crown to feet and back to the crown x 3.**</u>
This interval is the most fundamental one to build energy and eliminate fatigue. We use it near the end of the session, when one's energetic stores need to be nourished and consolidated.

STEP 9. SPEARMINT (use oil sparingly in this step, no more than 2-4 drops)

a. **Raindrop Spearmint Oil.** Holding bottle of Spearmint about six inches above the client's back, drop only 2-3 drops directly on the spine from sacrum to neck.

b. **3-6-12 Feathering Straight Up Spine.** Same procedure as Step 8b.

c. **Arched Feather Strokes (Angel Wings).** Same procedure as Step 8c.

d. **Full Length Strokes.** Same procedure as Step 8d.

STEP 10. HOT COMPRESS.

a. **Dry Towel.** Place a large dry bath towel covering client's back from hips to atlas.

b. **Hot Damp Towel.** Fold smaller towel into thirds, and roll into a cylinder. Then soak with hot water from the tap, wrung nearly dry, but still enough dampness to retain heat. Unroll the hot towel over the length of the spine rom neck to hips.
* Multiple Sclerosis (MS). For people with MS, use a cold pack, NOT a hot pack. A towel soaked in cold water will do. An ice pack is also okay.

c. **Another Dry Towel.** Lay another large towel over the compress to hold in heat.

d. <u>**Sound the High Full Moon Major 6th near the client's ears, circle around head, then move in a figure eight over the client, from crown to feet and back to the crown x 3.**</u>
Relax and know that the cleansing and release are perfect as the Full Moon energy brings the session to fullness.

e. **Sound the Ohm Octave to the sole of each foot at KI 1 (Gushing Spring) x 3, right foot first.**
The Ohm Octave brings feelings of comfort, completeness, and creates a sense of unity with All That Is. Thus ends our journey of healing with a Raindrop Technique session.

f. **Cooking the Client.** Oils will heat up and peak out in 5-8 minutes. If heat becomes too uncomfortable, apply V-6 or vegetable oil where needed. (See Note in Step 4.) Ask client to tell you when oils have cooled to a comfortable level.

g. **If Not Hot Enough.** If oils do not heat up with client, facilitator may place hands on back over the towel. NOTE: Because spearmint oil has been applied last, the client may experience what feels like coolness when, in fact, their back is warm.

STEP 11. REST & WATER

a. **Rest Quietly.** At this point client may wish to relax quietly for a few minutes. Whenever ready, they may sit up slowly with the facilitator standing nearby, being careful as they get off the massage table assisted by the facilitator.

b. **Drinking Water.** Have the client immediately drink a glass or bottle of good water and urge them to drink plenty of water for the next week.

STEP 12. RE-EVALUATION AND RE-MEASUREMENT.

a. **Measure Height Afterwards.** Re-measure client's height barefooted. Most will have grown from 1/4 to 1/2 inch. Those with severe spinal curvature may grow an inch or more. The benefits of Raindrop may not always include immediate growth but can be experienced by the receiver in other ways.

b. **Adjustments Continue for a Week.** A complete evaluation of the benefits received from Raindrop Technique may take several days to assess.

c. **Drink Lots of Water.** Remind the client to drink lots of water. The recommended amount is to divide their weight in pounds by two and drink that amount in ounces of pure (non-chlorinated) water every day. Additional

---

* These notes correspond to a 120-min DVD entitled *Raindrop Technique*. Available from CARE, RR 4 Box 646, Marble Hill, MO 63764
• (800) 758-8629 • or visit www.RaindropTraining.com.
Price: $29.95 + $9 s&h • Includes a set of notes

Additional Essential Oils Used in Raindrop Technique for Heart/Circulation

All of the Systems-specific Raindrop Technique protocol use Valor, oregano and thyme as the core three oils to open and close Raindrop Technique (EDOR, 4th Ed, page 299). Basil, marjoram, wintergreen, cypress and peppermint are replaced with oils more specific to the body system being treated. Details about the specific oils used to focus on the **Heart/Circulation** system are included below.

GOLDENROD (*Solidago canadensis*)--Family: Asteraceae (aster-daisy family), is a diuretic, anti-hypertensive. Contains 30-55% monoterpenes, 24-35% sesquiterpenes which may assist in restoring proper cellular programming to restore health and maintain wellness.

Slightly cooling, Goldenrod has an affinity with the Kidney and Spleen meridians. Its actions are similar to Cypress, in that it astringes fluid discharge that results from leakage of qi, such as urine, sweat, bedwetting, or diarrhea.

NUTMEG (*Myristica fragrans*)--Family: Myristicaceae (myrtle family), has potent anti-inflammatory (ORAC 158,100) and anticoagulant properties. Also used for its adrenal cortex-like activity to help support the adrenal glands for increased energy. Contains 55-80% monoterpenes which may assist in restoring proper cellular programming.

Warming Nutmeg has an affinity to the Liver, Spleen and Large Intestine meridians. It is useful for Deficient Spleen symptoms of chronic diarrhea, scant and painful menses and impotence. It will warm and regulate qi in the Middle Heater to assist with symptoms of nausea and vomiting.

AROMA LIFE® (contains helichrysum, ylang ylang, marjoram and cypress); improves cardiovascular, lymphatic and circulatory systems; lowers high blood pressure and reduces stress.

CYPRESS (*Cupressus sempervirens*) - Family: Cupressaceae (cypress family) is antimicrobial. Supportive of the circulatory and lymphatic systems. Stimulates the body's natural white corpuscle production. 76% monoterpenes and 14% sesquiterpenes which may assist in restoring proper cellular programming to restore health and maintain wellness.

Slightly cooling, Cypress has an affinity for Lung, Spleen and Kidney meridians. It astringes fluid discharge that results from leakage of qi, such as urine, sweat, or diarrhea. Cypress ascends Spleen qi to upbear prolapse, hemorrhoids and varicose veins. Finally, it is very helpful to clear Lung heat and assists the Kidney to grasp Lung qi in wheezing and bedwetting.

CLOVE (*Syzygium aromaticum*)--Family: myrtle family; anti-aging, cardiovascular disease, anticoagulant properties. Contains 70-85% phenols which cleanse cellular receptor sites.

Hot by nature, Clove has an affinity for the Spleen, Stomach and Kidney meridians. It can be used to warm the Kidneys to treat bone, teeth and impotence; warm the interior to expel Cold in the Stomach and Spleen to treat digestive problems and abdominal pain. Clove also improves thyroid and immune function by strengthening Deficient Spleen and Kidney qi.

Additional Intervals Used in Heart/Circulation Raindrop Technique

Fifth, 2:3
High Uranus/High Ohm - A Perfect Fifth, the Electrical Fifth; opens with the electrical charge of transformation, can shatter pre-existing conceptions and embodies the energy of freedom and independence. Mentally transformative, illuminating, inventive and break-through ideas. Uranus governs the electrical activity of the nervous system, and can calm and balance it.

Minor Seventh, 5:9
High Sun/Ohm - harsh but more distant, less emotional than the Minor 2nd (its inversion). Strong, warm energy, this interval is used near the completion of Raindrop to assist in deletion of old, redundant and useless information so changes can occur and a new order can be achieved.

Minor Sixth, 5:8
Venus/Ohm - mellow sense of longing; tonifies, nourishes beauty, harmony and creative passion but has a quality of inconstancy, desire and yearning for completion. Inversion of the Major Third (4th harmonic of overtone series). A Major Third plus a Minor Sixth creates an Octave. This interval is used for assisting with bone density and circulation.

Octave, 1:2
High Sun/Sonic Sun - very warming and energizing, bright sunshine on a cloudy day. This interval is used after the Ortho Ease rub to allow an interval of basking in the fullness of one's highest energy and well-being.

HEART & CIRCULATION
Vibrational Raindrop

Based on Raindrop Technique as Taught by D. Gary Young
At the Young Living Level I Training Conference in
Dallas, Texas, January 25-29, 2000
(From the CARE Raindrop Training Notes)

**The notes in Underlined Helvetica Bold are the tuning fork applications
to be done with the Heart/Circulation Raindrop Tuning Kit**

• **NOTE:** The person receiving oils is called the "client" or the "receiver." The person administering the oils is called the "facilitator." While this is the version of Raindrop taught by CARE Instructors, you may adapt the tuning forks to be used after the appropriate oils in different versions of Raindrop.

• **PRELIMINARIES:** Facilitator should trim nails as short as possible and file sharp corners and edges. Facilitator and client should both remove all metal, especially rings, bracelets, and watches.

STEP 1.   EVALUATION, PREPARATION AND PERMISSION.

a.   **Measure Height** of the client barefooted using a square box against a wall and sliding down to the head to assure a level measurement. This is not an essential part of raindrop, but is an objective demonstration of what often happens. Most people grow a little with a raindrop, but if one does not grow, that does not mean the raindrop has been ineffective or erroneously per formed.

b.   **Allergies, Sensitivities, Toxicity, etc.** Ask if client is prone to allergies, reactions to drugs or has developed any sensitizations to any sub stances. Mention to the client that allergic reactions to therapeutic grade essential oils are not possible, but sometimes there can be a detox reaction. Ask if they smoke or if they have ever engaged in occu pations exposing them to chemicals such as beauty shop, auto body, professional housecleaning, pesticides, herbicides, photo chemicals, environmental engineering, hospitals, etc.

c.   **Suggested Resources with Cleansing Information**: *Essential Oils Desk Reference*; *Reference Guide for Essential Oils*; *Healing for the Age of Enlightenment*.

d.   **Ask Permission.** After explaining the procedure to the client, ask permission to continue.

e.   **Bathroom:** Ask if client needs to use bathroom before you start.

f.   **Bodily Contact:** Once session begins, the facilitator should try to keep bodily contact with client at all times. When tuning forks are sounded around the client, the facilitator will need to break bodily contact to do this technique.

HEART & CIRCULATION

• HAVE CLIENT LIE FACE UP

STEP 2.   VALOR®.

a.   <u>Listen to the Ohm Unison x 3 (hold tuning forks to client's ears).</u>

b.   **Shoulders.** Place 3 drops of Valor on each shoulder. Hold for 5 minutes or more until a balance of energies is felt. Place your left hand on the left shoulder and your right hand on the right shoulder.

c.   **Soles of Feet.** Place 6 drops of Valor on the soles of each foot. Cross your arms so your right hand holds the right foot and your left hand holds the left foot. You will have to cross your arms to accomplish this.

d.   <u>Sound the Ohm Unison to the sole of each foot at KI 1 (Gushing Spring) and at KI 3 (Great Ravine) in the depression behind the inner ankle x 3, right foot first.</u> We begin the Raindrop journey from a firm, grounded place within. This interval deeply roots our core essence.

STEP 3.   VALOR, OREGANO, THYME, GOLDENROD, CLOVE, AROMALIFE, CYPRESS AND NUTMEG

a.   **Foot Vita Flex.** Vita Flex on each foot along spinal reflex points, coccyx to brain, starting with right foot. Each foot should be done with 2-3 drops per foot of each of the 8 oils in the order listed x 3.

b.   <u>Sound the Ohm Octave with Low Ohm at CV4 (Origin Pass) on the abdomen four finger-widths below the umbilicus, and Ohm at CV17 (Chest Center) in the center of the chest level with the 4th rib, x 3.</u> This interval creates a harmonic bridge and connection between the upper and lower body, further rooting our core energy.

• HAVE CLIENT ROLL OVER TO A FACE DOWN POSITION

STEP 4.   DUO: OREGANO AND THYME.*

a.   **Raindrop Oregano.** Holding bottle of Oregano about six inches above the client's back, drop 4-6 drops directly on the spine from sacrum to neck.

b.   **3-6-12 Feathering Straight Up Spine.** Feather stroke Oregano straight up the spine with a light touch using backs of fingernails gently brushing against client's skin. Start with 3" strokes alternately with each hand x 3 the length of the spine upwards to the atlas vertebra, then 6" strokes x 3, followed by 12" strokes x 3.

c.   **Thyme Raindrop.** Repeat a. & b. above for Thyme.

d.   **Feathering Straight to Sides.** After both Oregano and Thyme have been applied, starting at the sacrum, feather oils away from spine straight out nd down the sides x 3, then move up half-a-hand's width and repeat until you reach the neck and skull. Repeat this sacrum to atlas x 3.

e.   **Full Length Strokes.** Long feather strokes, both hands side by side, touching with back of nail tips only along both sides of the spine, sweep full length from sacrum to base of neck, fanning out and off the shoulders x 3.

f. **Sound the Solar 7th with the Low Ohm on GV2 (Low Back Shu) at base of sacrum and Sun fork on GV16 (Wind Mansion) on the back of the skull one inch above the posterior hairline.**
This interval assists the core Duo of Oregano and Thyme to "heat up" the cells and cleanse them for deletion of old, redundant and useless information. These two points achieve "cranial-sacral stillpoint" from which changes can occur and a new order can be achieved.

** **Important Note.** Some oils (particularly Oregano and Thyme) can cause heat when in contact with the skin and react with viruses, bacteria, and toxins. This is generally a good sign that the oils are seeking out and destroying harmful aliens that hibernate in the fatty tissue and lymph nodes along the spine. However, if at any time the heat becomes unpleasant for the client, apply V-6 or other vegetable oil where indicated. Relief should be immediate. Ask the client to tell you when and where this is needed throughout the Raindrop Technique session.*

STEP 5.   TRIO: GOLDENROD, CLOVE AND AROMALIFE
a. **Raindrop the Oils on the Back in the Order Given.** Follow steps a. & b. of STEP 4 above with Goldenrod, clove and AromaLife instead of Oregano and Thyme.
b. **Finger Circles.** After all three oils have been applied, apply your fingers to the laminar groove along one side of the spine, slowly progressing from sacrum to atlas, using four fingers of both hands together in a clockwise motion, pulling tissues away from spine with each circle. Then walk around table and go up other side. Alternate from side to side, right to left, until both sides have been done x 3. Apply AromaSiez® where tense muscles are discovered.
c. **Sound Zodiac 3rd wherever muscle knots are found at least x 3 at each location.**
If it is too painful to use the forks at the same location, then one fork can be placed on either side of the location of spasm.

*__Note on Additional Oils:__ At this point, before the finger circles, additional oils (such as Joy®, Frankincense, Release®, Relieve It®, Harmony®, Panaway®, etc.) may be applied if desired according to the wishes, needs, or special circumstances of the client. With each additional oil, drop them raindrop-style directly on the spine and then stroke them straight up the spine with the 3-6-12 feathering described in STEPS 4a and 4b. described above. **If other oils are added, sound the High Full Moon 6th near the client's ears, circle around head, then move in a figure eight over the client, from crown to feet and back to the crown x 3.** Relax and know that the cleansing and release are perfect and enjoy a sense of magic and fulfillment, with a pull towards healing that allows one's potential to manifest.*

STEP 6.   **CYPRESS.**

a.   **Sprinkle Cypress.** Sprinkle Cypress oil directly on the spine with a salt-shaker-like motion from sacrum to neck.

b.   **3-6-12 Feathering Straight Up Spine**. Feather straight up spine as described in STEP 4b. x 3.

c.   **Thumb Vita Flex.** Thumb Vita Flex along sides of spine from sacrum to atlas x 3.

d.   **Saw Maneuver & Skull-Pull.** Apply saw maneuver from sacrum to neck with three skull-pulls x 3.

e.   **Spine Stretch & Shake (or Quiver).** Apply two-handed spine stretch maneuver vibrating with a shaking or quivering motion perpendicular to the spine with each stretch, moving gradually upwards from sacrum to atlas. 3x.

f.   **Sound the Venus Minor 6th on the Huato Jiaji points up the spine from sacrum to base of skull. The Huato Jiaji points are found on either side of the spine between the vertebrae. Then hold both forks together at GV20 (Hundred Convergences) in the depression at the crown of the head and** also **near the ears to allow client to hear the interval.**
This interval is used for assisting with bone density and circulation.

STEP 7.   **ORTHO EASE®.**

a.   **Apply Ortho Ease Oil.** Dispense oil generously onto palms first, then apply over the entire back, spreading it with flat palms of the hands in clockwise circular movements from hips to neck, cross over, and then back down to the hips. Repeat x 3. A free style anointing without structure or counting may be done. Include attention of the shoulder blades, neck, trapezium muscles, and places that are tight or sore. Ask client if they have any particular requests in this regard.

b.   **(Optional) Rest** Quietly rest face down for 4-5 minutes. Cover with sheet to keep client warm and comfortable, if necessary. Apply more Ortho Ease as needed, repeating step 7a.

c.   **Indian Rub.** Perform see-saw rub maneuver across the spine progressing from sacrum to neck and from neck to sacrum, up and down the back at least x 3. Except for step 7a. above, this is the only procedure performed both up and down the back. All others are done up only, from sacrum to neck.

d.   **Sound the High Sun/Sonic Sun Octave near the client's ears, circle around head, then move in a figure eight over the client, from crown to feet and back to the crown x 3.**
This interval is used after the Ortho Ease rub to allow an interval of basking in the fullness of one's highest energy and well-being.

STEP 8.   VALOR®.
a.   **Sprinkle Valor.** Sprinkle Valor oil directly on the spine with salt-shaker-like motion from sacrum to neck. Valor is a mild oil blend that does not get hot and can be applied generously.
b.   **3-6-12 Feathering Straight Up Spine.** Feather straight up spine as described STEP 4b. x 3.
c.   **Arched Feather Strokes (Angel Wings).** Feather with backs of fingernails in a curved fanning motion arched up and out to sides in 3" strokes (3x), 6" strokes (3x) and 12" strokes (3x).
d.   **Full Length Strokes.** Long feather strokes from sacrum up to and off of the shoulders as described in STEP 4e. 3x.
e.   **<u>Sound the High Earth Day 5th near the client's ears, circle around head, then move in a figure eight over the client, from crown to feet and back to the crown x 3.</u>**
Strong, warm energy, this interval is used near the completion of Raindrop to assist in deletion of old, redundant and useless information so changes can occur and a new order can be achieved.

STEP 9.   NUTMEG (use oil sparingly in this step, no more than 2-4 drops)
a.   **Raindrop Nutmeg Oil.** Holding bottle of Nutmeg about six inches above the client's back, drop only 2-3 drops directly on the spine from sacrum to neck.
b.   **3-6-12 Feathering Straight Up Spine.** Same procedure as Step 8b.
c.   **Arched Feather Strokes (Angel Wings).** Same procedure as Step 8c.
d.   **Full Length Strokes.** Same procedure as Step 8d.

STEP 10.   HOT COMPRESS.
a.   **Dry Towel.** Place large dry bath towel covering client's back from hips to atlas.
b.   **Hot Damp Towel.** Fold smaller towel into thirds, and roll into a cylinder. Then soak with hot water from the tap, wrung nearly dry, but still enough dampness to retain heat. Unroll the hot towel over the length of the spine from neck to hips.
     * **Multiple Sclerosis (MS).** For people with MS, use a cold pack, NOT a hot pack. A towel soaked in cold water will do. An ice pack is also okay.
c.   **Another Dry Towel.** Lay another large towel over the compress to hold in heat.
d.   **<u>Sound the High Uranus 5th near the client's ears, circle around head, then move in a figure eight over the client, from crown to feet and back to the crown x 3.</u>**
Uranus governs the electrical activity of the nervous system, and can calm and balance it.
e.   **<u>Sound the Ohm Octave to the sole of each foot at KI 1 (Gushing Spring) x 3, right foot first.</u>** The Ohm Octave brings feelings of comfort, completeness, and creates a sense of unity with All That Is. Thus ends our journey of healing with a Raindrop Technique session.

f.   **Cooking the Client.** Oils will heat up and peak out in 5-8 minutes. If heat becomes too uncomfortable, apply V-6 or vegetable oil where needed. (See Note in Step 4.) Ask client to tell you when oils have cooled to a comfortable level.

g.   **If Not Hot Enough.** If oils do not heat up with client, facilitator may place hands on back over the towel. NOTE: Because nutmeg oil has been applied last, the client may experience some confusion as to whether their back feels warm or cool.

STEP 11.   REST & WATER

a.   **Rest Quietly**. At this point client may wish to relax quietly for a few minutes. Whenever ready, they may sit up slowly with the facilitator standing nearby, being careful as they get off the massage table assisted by the facilitator.

b.   **Drinking Water.** Have the client immediately drink a glass or bottle of good water and urge them to drink plenty of water for the next week.

STEP 12.   RE-EVALUATION AND RE-MEASUREMENT.

a.   **Measure Height Afterwards**. Re-measure client's height barefooted. Most will have grown from 1/4 to 1/2 inch. Those with severe spinal curvature may grow an inch or more. The benefits of Raindrop may not always include immediate growth but can be experienced by the receiver in other ways.

b.   **Adjustments Continue for a Week.** A complete evaluation of the benefits received from Raindrop Technique may take several days to assess.

c.   **Drink Lots of Water.** Remind the client to drink lots of water. The recommended amount is to divide their weight in pounds by two and drink that amount in ounces of pure (non-chlorinated) water every day. Additional

---

* These notes correspond to a 120-min DVD entitled *Raindrop Technique*.
Available from CARE, RR 4 Box 646, Marble Hill, MO 63764
• (800) 758-8629 • or visit www.RaindropTraining.com.
Price: $29.95 + $9 s&h • Includes a set of notes

Additional Essential Oils Used
in Raindrop for Female Hormone Balance

All of the Systems-specific Raindrop Technique protocol use Valor, oregano and thyme as the core three oils to open and close Raindrop Technique (EDOR, 4th Ed, page 299). Basil, marjoram, wintergreen, cypress and peppermint are replaced with oils more specific to the body system being treated. Details about the specific oils used to focus on the **Hormone Balance - Female system** are included below.

DRAGON TIME® (contains clary sage, blue yarrow, lavender, jasmine, fennel and marjoram); relieves PMS symptoms as well as cramping, irregular periods and mood swings caused by hormonal imbalance.

FLEABANE (*Conyza canadensis*)--Family: Asteraceae or Compositae (daisy); is hormone-like, antirheumatic, antispasmodic and a cardiovascular dilator. Contains 63-83% monoterpenes.

With an affinity for the Kidney, Lung and Spleen meridians, Fleabane is cool in nature. It expels Hot Phlegm and Nourishes Yin, so use it for bronchitis and fevers, as well as a diuretic for edema.

ENDO FLEX® (contains spearmint, sage, geranium, myrtle, German Chamomile and nutmeg); amplifies metabolism and vitality, and creates hormonal balance.

CLARY SAGE (*Salvia sclarea*)--Family: Lamiaceae (mint); naturally raises estrogen and progesterone levels, antidiabetic, antifungal, cholesterol-reducing. Very calming and stress-relieving; enhances dreams. Contains 50-78% esters, up to 27% alcohols and up to 14% sesquiterpenes.

Cooling Clary Sage has an affinity for the Liver, Heart and Kidney meridians. It cools Heat in the Blood and Empty Fire with symptoms of night sweats, hot flashes and insomnia. Tonifies Heart Blood and Yin deficiency to resolve anxiety and insomnia.

PEPPERMINT (*Mentha piperita*) CT menthol - Family: Lamiaceae supports digestive system, respiratory system, and nervous system. Has been used for headaches. Research has shown that inhaling peppermint improves concentration and mental retention. Detoxing to the liver. A synergistic oil that supports and improves the beneficial actions of other oils used in conjunction. High in phenolics, but contains 9% sesquiterpenes.

Peppermint has an affinity for the Lung and Liver meridians with its cooling energy. Clears Wind Heat of headaches, fever, sore throat, and dry cough, as well as regulates Liver qi to promote menstruation, and decongest the Liver/PMS. It also promotes the movement of Wei qi.

Additional Intervals Used in
Raindrop Technique for Female Hormone Balance

Minor Second, 15:16

High Saturn/High Ohm - semitone and somewhat dissonant, supports the formation of new boundaries and structures. The Minor Second is the most dissonant of the intervals, and Saturn/Ohm is more dissonant than Mars/Ohm. They both represent the applications of energy toward the manifestation of material form, in other words creating matter from spirit. Twin pillars of evolution on the material and spiritual planes. We use this interval near the end of the Raindrop session to consolidate the endocrine and hormonal balancing that has begun with Raindrop.

Fifth, 2:3

New Moon/Ohm - calming, relaxing, opening. The New Moon 5th is dispersive for emotional issues, while the Earth Day 5th is better suited to gather and strengthen energy. This interval produces openings on the physical, emotional, and spiritual levels.

Minor Sixth, 5:8

High Venus/High Ohm - mellow sense of longing; tonifies, nourishes beauty, harmony and creative passion but has a quality of inconstancy, desire and yearning for completion. Inversion of the Major Third (4th harmonic of overtone series). A Major Third plus a Minor Sixth creates an Octave. This interval can assist with reproductive problems and menopausal hormonal imbalances. Relax and know that the cleansing and release are perfect as the Venus energy brings the session to fullness.

HORMONE BALANCE - FEMALE
Vibrational Raindrop

Based on Raindrop Technique as Taught by D. Gary Young
At the Young Living Level I Training Conference in
Dallas, Texas, January 25-29, 2000
(From the CARE Raindrop Training Notes)

**The notes in Underlined Helvetica Bold are the tuning fork applications
to be done with the Hormone Balance - Female Raindrop Tuning Kit**

• **NOTE:**   The person receiving oils is called the "client" or the "receiver." The person administering the oils is called the "facilitator." While this is the version of Raindrop taught by CARE Instructors, you may adapt the tuning forks to be used after the appropriate oils in different versions of Raindrop.

• **PRELIMINARIES:** Facilitator should trim nails as short as possible and file sharp corners and edges. Facilitator and client should both remove all metal, especially rings, bracelets, and watches.

STEP 1.   EVALUATION, PREPARATION AND PERMISSION.

a.   **Measure Height** of the client barefooted using a square box against a wall and sliding down to the head to assure a level measurement. This is not an essential part of raindrop, but is an objective demonstration of what often happens. Most people grow a little with a raindrop, but if one does not grow, that does not mean the raindrop has been ineffective or erroneously per   formed.

b.   **Allergies, Sensitivities, Toxicity, etc.** Ask if client is prone to allergies, reactions to drugs or has developed any sensitizations to any sub stances. Mention to the client that allergic reactions to therapeutic grade essential oils are not possible, but sometimes there can be a detox reaction. Ask if they smoke or if they have ever engaged in occu pations exposing them to chemicals such as beauty shop, auto body, professional housecleaning, pesticides, herbicides, photo chemicals, environmental engineering, hospitals, etc.

c.   **Suggested Resources with Cleansing Information**: *Essential Oils Desk Reference*; *Reference Guide for Essential Oils*; *Healing for the Age of Enlightenment*.

d.   **Ask Permission.** After explaining the procedure to the client, ask permission to continue.

e.   **Bathroom:** Ask if client needs to use bathroom before you start.

f.   **Bodily Contact:** Once session begins, the facilitator should try to keep bodily contact with client at all times. When tuning forks are sounded around the client, the facilitator will need to break bodily contact to do this technique.

• **HAVE CLIENT LIE FACE UP**

STEP 2.   VALOR®.

a.   <u>Listen to the Ohm Unison x 3 (hold tuning forks to client's ears).</u>

b.   **Shoulders.** Place 3 drops of Valor on each shoulder. Hold for 5 minutes or more until a balance of energies is felt. Place your left hand on the left shoulder and your right hand on the right shoulder.

c.   **Soles of Feet.** Place 6 drops of Valor on the soles of each foot. Cross your arms so your right hand holds the right foot and your left hand holds the left foot. You will have to cross your arms to accomplish this.

d.   <u>Sound the Ohm Unison to the sole of each foot at KI 1 (Gushing Spring) and at KI 3 (Great Ravine) in the depression behind the inner ankle x 3, right foot first.</u> We begin the Raindrop journey from a firm, grounded place within. This interval deeply roots our core essence.

STEP 3.   VALOR, OREGANO, THYME, DRAGON TIME, FLEABANE, ENDOFLEX, CLARY SAGE, and PEPPERMINT.

a.   **Foot Vita Flex.** Vita Flex on each foot along spinal reflex points, coccyx to brain, starting with right foot. Each foot should be done with 2-3 drops per foot of each of the 8 oils in the order listed x 3.

b.   <u>Sound the Ohm Octave with Low Ohm at CV4 (Origin Pass) on the abdomen four finger-widths below the umbilicus, and Ohm at CV17 (Chest Center) in the center of the chest level with the 4th rib, x 3.</u> This interval creates a harmonic bridge and connection between the upper and lower body, further rooting our core energy.

• **HAVE CLIENT ROLL OVER TO A FACE DOWN POSITION**

STEP 4.   DUO: OREGANO AND THYME.*

a.   **Raindrop Oregano.** Holding bottle of Oregano about six inches above the client's back, drop 4-6 drops directly on the spine from sacrum to neck.

b.   **3-6-12 Feathering Straight Up Spine.** Feather stroke Oregano straight up the spine with a light touch using backs of fingernails gently brushing against client's skin. Start with 3" strokes alternately with each hand x 3 the length of the spine upwards to the atlas vertebra, then 6" strokes x 3, followed by 12" strokes x 3.

c.   **Thyme Raindrop.** Repeat a. & b. above for Thyme.

d.   **Feathering Straight to Sides.** After both Oregano and Thyme have been applied, starting at the sacrum, feather oils away from spine straight out nd down the sides x 3, then move up half-a-hand's width and repeat until you reach the neck and skull. Repeat this sacrum to atlas x 3.

e.   **Full Length Strokes.** Long feather strokes, both hands side by side, touching with back of nail tips only along both sides of the spine, sweep full length from sacrum to base of neck, fanning out and off the shoulders x 3.

f.   **Sound the Solar 7th with the Low Ohm on GV2 (Low Back Shu) at base of sacrum and Sun fork on GV16 (Wind Mansion) on the back of the skull one inch above the posterior hairline.**
This interval assists the core Duo of Oregano and Thyme to "heat up" the cells and cleanse them for deletion of old, redundant and useless information. These two points achieve "cranial-sacral stillpoint" from which changes can occur and a new order can be achieved.

** **Important Note.**   Some oils (particularly Oregano and Thyme) can cause heat when in contact with the skin and react with viruses, bacteria, and toxins. This is generally a good sign that the oils are seeking out and destroying harmful aliens that hibernate in the fatty tissue and lymph nodes along the spine. However, if at any time the heat becomes unpleasant for the client, apply V-6 or other vegetable oil where indicated. Relief should be immediate. Ask the client to tell you when and where this is needed throughout the Raindrop Technique session.*

STEP 5.   TRIO: DRAGON TIME, FLEABANE, AND ENDOFLEX
a.   **Raindrop the Oils on the Back in the Order Given.** Follow steps
a. & b. of STEP 4 above with Dragon Time, Fleabane, and Endoflex instead of Oregano and Thyme.
b.   **Finger Circles.** After all three oils have been applied, apply your fingers to the laminar groove along one side of the spine, slowly progressing from sacrum to atlas, using four fingers of both hands together in a clockwise motion, pulling tissues away from spine with each circle. Then walk around table and go up other side. Alternate from side to side, right to left, until both sides have been done x 3. Apply AromaSiez® where tense muscles are discovered.
c.   **Sound Zodiac 3rd wherever muscle knots are found at least x 3 at each location.**
If it is too painful to use the forks at the same location, then one fork can be placed on either side of the location of spasm.

Note on Additional Oils: *At this point, before the finger circles, additional oils (such as Joy®, Frankincense, Release®, Relieve It®, Harmony®, Panaway®, etc.) may be applied if desired according to the wishes, needs, or special circumstances of the client. With each additional oil, drop them raindrop-style directly on the spine and then stroke them straight up the spine with the 3-6-12 feathering described in STEPS 4a and 4b. described above.* **If other oils are added, sound the High Full Moon 6th near the client's ears, circle around head, then move in a figure eight over the client, from crown to feet and back to the crown x 3.** *Relax and know that the cleansing and release are perfect and enjoy a sense of magic and fulfillment, with a pull towards healing that allows one's potential to manifest.*

STEP 6.   CLARY SAGE.

a.   **Sprinkle Clary Sage.** Sprinkle Clary Sage oil directly on the spine with a salt-shaker-like motion from sacrum to neck.

b.   **3-6-12 Feathering Straight Up Spine.** Feather straight up spine as described in STEP 4b. x 3.

c.   **Thumb Vita Flex.** Thumb Vita Flex along sides of spine from sacrum to atlas x 3.

d.   **Saw Maneuver & Skull-Pull.** Apply saw maneuver from sacrum to neck with three skull-pulls x 3.

e.   **Spine Stretch & Shake (or Quiver).** Apply two-handed spine stretch maneuver vibrating with a shaking or quivering motion perpendicular to the spine with each stretch, moving gradually upwards from sacrum to atlas. 3x.

f.   **Sound the New Moon 5th on the Huato Jiaji points up the spine from sacrum to base of skull. The Huato Jiaji points are found on either side of the spine between the vertebrae. Then hold both forks together at GV20 (Hundred Convergences) in the depression at the crown of the head and also near the ears to allow client to hear the interval.**
      This interval produces openings on the physical, emotional, and spiritual levels.

STEP 7.   ORTHO EASE®.

a.   **Apply Ortho Ease Oil.** Dispense oil generously onto palms first, then apply over the entire back, spreading it with flat palms of the hands in clockwise circular movements from hips to neck, cross over, and then back down to the hips. Repeat x 3. A free style anointing without structure or counting may be done. Include attention of the shoulder blades, neck, trapezium muscles, and places that are tight or sore. Ask client if they have any particular requests in this regard.

b.   **(Optional) Rest Quietly** rest face down for 4-5 minutes. Cover with sheet to keep client warm and comfortable, if necessary. Apply more Ortho Ease as needed, repeating step 7a.

c.   **Indian Rub.** Perform see-saw rub maneuver across the spine progressing from sacrum to neck and from neck to sacrum, up and down the back at least x 3. Except for step 7a. above, this is the only procedure performed both up and down the back. All others are done up only, from sacrum to neck.

d.   **Sound the High Jupiter 4th near the client's ears, circle around head, then move in a figure eight over the client, from crown to feet and back to the crown x 3.**
      The major energetic work of a Raindrop session has been done, and we relax for a few minutes to enjoy the bounty of it all.

STEP 8.   VALOR®.

a.   **Sprinkle Valor.** Sprinkle Valor oil directly on the spine with salt-shaker-like motion from sacrum to neck. Valor is a mild oil blend that does not get hot and can be applied generously.

b.   **3-6-12 Feathering Straight Up Spine.** Feather straight up spine as described STEP 4b. x 3.

c.   **Arched Feather Strokes (Angel Wings).** Feather with backs of fingernails in a curved fanning motion arched up and out to sides in 3" strokes (3x), 6" strokes (3x) and 12" strokes (3x).

d.   **Full Length Strokes.** Long feather strokes from sacrum up to and off of the shoulders as described in STEP 4e. 3x.

e.   <u>**Sound the High Saturn minor 2nd near the client's ears, circle around head, then move in a figure eight over the client, from crown to feet and back to the crown x 3.**</u>
We use this interval near the end of the Raindrop session to consolidate the endocrine and hormonal balancing that has begun with Raindrop.

STEP 9.   PEPPERMINT (use oil sparingly in this step, no more than 2-4 drops)

a.   **Raindrop Peppermint Oil.** Holding bottle of Peppermint about six inches above the client's back, drop only 2-3 drops directly on the spine from sacrum to neck.

b.   **3-6-12 Feathering Straight Up Spine.** Same procedure as Step 8b.

c.   **Arched Feather Strokes (Angel Wings)**. Same procedure as Step 8c.

d.   **Full Length Strokes.** Same procedure as Step 8d.

STEP 10.   HOT COMPRESS.

a.   **Dry Towel.** Place large dry bath towel covering client's back from hips to atlas.

b.   **Hot Damp Towel**. Fold smaller towel into thirds, and roll into a cylinder. Then soak with hot water from the tap, wrung nearly dry, but still enough dampness to retain heat. Unroll the hot towel over the length of the spine from neck to hips.
* **Multiple Sclerosis (MS)**. For people with MS, use a cold pack, NOT a hot pack. A towel soaked in cold water will do. An ice pack is also okay.

c.   **Another Dry Towel.** Lay another large towel over the compress to hold in heat.

d.   <u>**Sound the High Venus Minor 6th near the client's ears, circle around head, then move in a figure eight over the client, from crown to feet and back to the crown x 3.**</u>
This interval can assist with reproductive problems and menopausal hormonal imbalances. Relax and know that the cleansing and release are perfect as the Venus energy brings the session to fullness.

e. **Sound the Ohm Octave to the sole of each foot at KI 1 (Gushing Spring) x 3, right foot first.**
The Ohm Octave brings feelings of comfort, completeness, and creates a sense of unity with All That Is. Thus ends our journey of healing with a Raindrop Technique session.

f. **Cooking the Client**. Oils will heat up and peak out in 5-8 minutes. If heat becomes too uncomfortable, apply V-6 or vegetable oil where needed. (See Note in Step 4.) Ask client to tell you when oils have cooled to a comfortable level.

g. **If Not Hot Enough**. If oils do not heat up with client, facilitator may place hands on back over the towel. NOTE: Because peppermint oil has been applied last, the client may experience what feels like coolness when, in fact, their back is warm.

STEP 11. REST & WATER
a. **Rest Quietly**. At this point client may wish to relax quietly for a few minutes. Whenever ready, they may sit up slowly with the facilitator standing nearby, being careful as they get off the massage table assisted by the facilitator.

b. **Drinking Water.** Have the client immediately drink a glass or bottle of good water and urge them to drink plenty of water for the next week.

STEP 12. RE-EVALUATION AND RE-MEASUREMENT.
a. **Measure Height Afterwards**. Re-measure client's height barefooted. Most will have grown from 1/4 to 1/2 inch. Those with severe spinal curvature may grow an inch or more. The benefits of Raindrop may not always include immediate growth but can be experienced by the receiver in other ways.

b. **Adjustments Continue for a Week.** A complete evaluation of the benefits received from Raindrop Technique may take several days to assess.

c. **Drink Lots of Water.** Remind the client to drink lots of water. The recommended amount is to divide their weight in pounds by two and drink that amount in ounces of pure (non-chlorinated) water every day. Additional

---

* These notes correspond to a 120-min DVD entitled *Raindrop Technique*.
Available from CARE, RR 4 Box 646, Marble Hill, MO 63764
• (800) 758-8629 • or visit www.RaindropTraining.com.
Price: $29.95 + $9 s&h • Includes a set of notes

Additional Essential Oils Used
in Raindrop for Male Hormone Balance

All of the Systems-specific Raindrop Technique protocol use Valor, oregano and thyme as the core three oils to open and close Raindrop Technique (EDOR, 4th Ed, page 299). Basil, marjoram, wintergreen, cypress and peppermint are replaced with oils more specific to the body system being treated. Details about the specific oils used to focus on the **Hormone Balance - Male** system are included below.

LAVENDER (*Lavandula angustifolia*)--Family: Lamiacea (mint); relaxant, combats excess sebum on skin, calming both physically and emotionally. Contains 30-58% alcohols, 26-52% esters.

Cooling Lavendar has an affinity for the Lung, Liver, and Pericardium meridians. Use it for Liver Qi Stagnation to promote the smooth flow of Liver qi and resolve headaches, muscle spasms and tightness. Also indicated to Calm the Shen and resolves symptoms of irritability, restlessness and high blood pressure (Liver and Heart Fire).

BLUE YARROW (*Achillea millefolium*)--Family: Asteraceae or Compositae (daisy); considered sacred by the Chinese who recognize the harmony of the Yin and Yang energies within it; where heaven meets earth.

Yarrow is cold in nature with an affinity for the Lung, Liver and Spleen channels. It is useful for Liver Qi Stagnation symptoms of muscle spasm, wind-bi (radiating pain), indecisiveness and itching skin. It will also release the Exterior by promoting diaphoresis and expelling Phlegm.

MISTER® (contains blue yarrow, sage, myrtle fennel, lavender and peppermint); helps to decongest the prostate and promote greater male hormonal balance.

MYRTLE (*Myrtus communis*)--Family: Myrtaceae (myrtle); normalizes hormonal imbalances, thyroid problems, prostate problems, muscle spasms. Contains 31-48% oxides, 30-45% monoterpenes.

Dry and cool, Myrtle clears Lung Heat and astringes leakage of qi and Blood such as sweating, bleeding, diarrhea and hemorrhoids. It is calming as a nervine.

PEPPERMINT (*Mentha piperita*) CT menthol - Family: Lamiaceae supports digestive system, respiratory system, and nervous system. Has been used for headaches. Research has shown that inhaling peppermint improves concentration and mental retention. Detoxing to the liver. A synergistic oil that supports and improves the beneficial actions of other oils used in conjunction. High in phenolics, but contains 9% sesquiterpenes.

Peppermint has an affinity for the Lung and Liver meridians with its cooling energy. Clears Wind Heat of headaches, fever, sore throat, and dry cough. Peppermint also regulates Liver qi which, in women, promotes menstruation, and decongest the Liver/PMS. It also promotes the movement of Wei qi.

Additional Intervals Used in Raindrop for Male Hormone Balance

Minor Second, 15:16

High Saturn/High Ohm - semitone and somewhat dissonant, supports the formation of new boundaries and structures. The Minor Second is the most dissonant of the intervals, and Saturn/Ohm is more dissonant than Mars/Ohm. They both represent the applications of energy toward the manifestation of material form, in other words creating matter from spirit. Twin pillars of evolution on the material and spiritual planes. We use this interval near the end of the Raindrop session to consolidate the endocrine and hormonal balancing that has begun with Raindrop.

Fifth, 2:3

New Moon/Ohm - calming, relaxing, opening. The New Moon 5th is dispersive for emotional issues, while the Earth Day 5th is better suited to gather and strengthen energy. This interval produces openings on the physical, emotional, and spiritual levels.

Minor Sixth, 5:8

High Venus/High Ohm - mellow sense of longing; tonifies, nourishes beauty, harmony and creative passion but has a quality of inconstancy, desire and yearning for completion. Inversion of the Major Third (4th harmonic of overtone series). A Major Third plus a Minor Sixth creates an Octave. This interval can assist with reproductive problems and menopausal hormonal imbalances. Relax and know that the cleansing and release are perfect as the Venus energy brings the session to fullness.

HORMONE BALANCE - MALE
Vibrational Raindrop

Based on Raindrop Technique as Taught by D. Gary Young
At the Young Living Level I Training Conference in
Dallas, Texas, January 25-29, 2000
(From the CARE Raindrop Training Notes)

The notes in Underlined Helvetica Bold are the tuning fork applications to be done with the Hormone Balance - Male Raindrop Tuning Kit

• **NOTE:** The person receiving oils is called the "client" or the "receiver." The person administering the oils is called the "facilitator." While this is the version of Raindrop taught by CARE Instructors, you may adapt the tuning forks to be used after the appropriate oils in different versions of Raindrop.

• **PRELIMINARIES:** Facilitator should trim nails as short as possible and file sharp corners and edges. Facilitator and client should both remove all metal, especially rings, bracelets, and watches.

STEP 1.   EVALUATION, PREPARATION AND PERMISSION.

a.   **Measure Height** of the client barefooted using a square box against a wall and sliding down to the head to assure a level measurement. This is not an essential part of raindrop, but is an objective demonstration of what often happens. Most people grow a little with a raindrop, but if one does not grow, that does not mean the raindrop has been ineffective or erroneously per formed.

b.   **Allergies, Sensitivities, Toxicity, etc.** Ask if client is prone to allergies, reactions to drugs or has developed any sensitizations to any sub stances. Mention to the client that allergic reactions to therapeutic grade essential oils are not possible, but sometimes there can be a detox reaction. Ask if they smoke or if they have ever engaged in occu pations exposing them to chemicals such as beauty shop, auto body, professional housecleaning, pesticides, herbicides, photo chemicals, environmental engineering, hospitals, etc.

c.   **Suggested Resources with Cleansing Information**: *Essential Oils Desk Reference*; *Reference Guide for Essential Oils*; *Healing for the Age of Enlightenment.*

d.   **Ask Permission.** After explaining the procedure to the client, ask permission to continue.

e.   **Bathroom:** Ask if client needs to use bathroom before you start.

f.   **Bodily Contact:** Once session begins, the facilitator should try to keep bodily contact with client at all times. When tuning forks are sounded around the client, the facilitator will need to break bodily contact to do this technique.

• HAVE CLIENT LIE FACE UP

STEP 2.   VALOR®.

a. <u>**Listen to the Ohm Unison x 3 (hold tuning forks to client's ears).**</u>

b. **Shoulders.** Place 3 drops of Valor on each shoulder. Hold for 5 minutes or more until a balance of energies is felt. Place your left hand on the left shoulder and your right hand on the right shoulder.

c. **Soles of Feet.** Place 6 drops of Valor on the soles of each foot. Cross your arms so your right hand holds the right foot and your left hand holds the left foot. You will have to cross your arms to accomplish this.

d. <u>**Sound the Ohm Unison to the sole of each foot at KI 1 (Gushing Spring) and at KI 3 (Great Ravine) in the depression behind the inner ankle x 3, right foot first.**</u> We begin the Raindrop journey from a firm, grounded place within. This interval deeply roots our core essence.

STEP 3.   VALOR, OREGANO, THYME, LAVENDER, BLUE YARROW, MISTER® , MYRTLE and PEPPERMINT.

a. **Foot Vita Flex.** Vita Flex on each foot along spinal reflex points, coccyx to brain, starting with right foot. Each foot should be done with 2-3 drops per foot of each of the 8 oils in the order listed x 3.

b. <u>**Sound the Ohm Octave with Low Ohm at CV4 (Origin Pass) on the abdomen four finger-widths below the umbilicus, and Ohm at CV17 (Chest Center) in the center of the chest level with the 4th rib, x 3.**</u>
This interval creates a harmonic bridge and connection between the upper and lower body, further rooting our core energy.

• HAVE CLIENT ROLL OVER TO A FACE DOWN POSITION

STEP 4.   DUO: OREGANO AND THYME.*

a. **Raindrop Oregano.** Holding bottle of Oregano about six inches above the client's back, drop 4-6 drops directly on the spine from sacrum to neck.

b. **3-6-12 Feathering Straight Up Spine.** Feather stroke Oregano straight up the spine with a light touch using backs of fingernails gently brushing against client's skin. Start with 3" strokes alternately with each hand x 3 the length of the spine upwards to the atlas vertebra, then 6" strokes x 3, followed by 12" strokes x 3.

c. **Thyme Raindrop.** Repeat a. & b. above for Thyme.

d. **Feathering Straight to Sides.** After both Oregano and Thyme have been applied, starting at the sacrum, feather oils away from spine straight out nd down the sides x 3, then move up half-a-hand's width and repeat until you reach the neck and skull. Repeat this sacrum to atlas x 3.

e. **Full Length Strokes.** Long feather strokes, both hands side by side, touching with back of nail tips only along both sides of the spine, sweep full length from sacrum to base of neck, fanning out and off the shoulders x 3.

f. <u>**Sound the Solar 7th with the Low Ohm on GV2 (Low Back Shu) at base of sacrum and Sun fork on GV16 (Wind Mansion) on the back of the skull one inch above the posterior hairline.**</u>

This interval assists the core Duo of Oregano and Thyme to "heat up" the cells and cleanse them for deletion of old, redundant and useless information. These two points achieve "cranial-sacral stillpoint" from which changes can occur and a new order can be achieved.

__Important Note.__ Some oils (particularly Oregano and Thyme) can cause heat when in contact with the skin and react with viruses, bacteria, and toxins. This is generally a good sign that the oils are seeking out and destroying harmful aliens that hibernate in the fatty tissue and lymph nodes along the spine. However, if at any time the heat becomes unpleasant for the client, apply V-6 or other vegetable oil where indicated. Relief should be immediate. Ask the client to tell you when and where this is needed throughout the Raindrop Technique session.

STEP 5.   TRIO: LAVENDER, BLUE YARROW, AND MISTER

a. **Raindrop the Oils on the Back in the Order Given.** Follow steps a. & b. of STEP 4 above with Lavender, Blue Yarrow and Mister instead of Oregano and Thyme.

b. **Finger Circles.** After all three oils have been applied, apply your fingers to the laminar groove along one side of the spine, slowly progressing from sacrum to atlas, using four fingers of both hands together in a clockwise motion, pulling tissues away from spine with each circle. Then walk around table and go up other side. Alternate from side to side, right to left, until both sides have been done x 3. Apply AromaSiez® where tense muscles are discovered.

c. <u>**Sound Zodiac 3rd wherever muscle knots are found at least x 3 at each location.**</u>

If it is too painful to use the forks at the same location, then one fork can be placed on either side of the location of spasm.

__Note on Additional Oils:__ At this point, before the finger circles, additional oils (such as Joy®, Frankincense, Release®, Relieve It®, Harmony®, Panaway®, etc.) may be applied if desired according to the wishes, needs, or special circumstances of the client. With each additional oil, drop them raindrop-style directly on the spine and then stroke them straight up the spine with the 3-6-12 feathering described in STEPS 4a and 4b. described above. __If other oils are added, sound the High Full Moon 6th near the client's ears, circle around head, then move in a figure eight over the client, from crown to feet and back to the crown x 3.__ Relax and know that the cleansing and release are perfect and enjoy a sense of magic and fulfillment, with a pull towards healing that allows one's potential to manifest.

STEP 6.   MYRTLE.

a.   **Sprinkle Myrtle**. Sprinkle Myrtle oil directly on the spine with a salt-shaker-like motion from sacrum to neck.

b.   **3-6-12 Feathering Straight Up Spine.** Feather straight up spine as described in STEP 4b. x 3.

c.   Thumb Vita Flex. Thumb Vita Flex along sides of spine from sacrum to atlas x 3.

d.   **Saw Maneuver & Skull-Pull.** Apply saw maneuver from sacrum to neck with three skull-pulls x 3.

e.   **Spine Stretch & Shake (or Quiver).** Apply two-handed spine stretch maneuver vibrating with a shaking or quivering motion perpendicular to the spine with each stretch, moving gradually upwards from sacrum to atlas. 3x.

f.   <u>**Sound the New Moon 5th on the Huato Jiaji points up the spine from sacrum to base of skull. The Huato Jiaji points are found on either side of the spine between the vertebrae. Then hold both forks together at GV20 (Hundred Convergences) in the depression at the crown of the head and also near the ears to allow client to hear the interval.**</u>
This interval produces openings on the physical, emotional, and spiritual levels.

STEP 7.   ORTHO EASE®.

a.   **Apply Ortho Ease Oil.** Dispense oil generously onto palms first, then apply over the entire back, spreading it with flat palms of the hands in clockwise circular movements from hips to neck, cross over, and then back down to the hips. Repeat x 3. A free style anointing without structure or counting may be done. Include attention of the shoulder blades, neck, trapezium muscles, and places that are tight or sore. Ask client if they have any particular requests in this regard.

b.   **(Optional) Rest Quietly** rest face down for 4-5 minutes. Cover with sheet to keep client warm and comfortable, if necessary. Apply more Ortho Ease as needed, repeating step 7a.

c.   **Indian Rub.** Perform see-saw rub maneuver across the spine progressing from sacrum to neck and from neck to sacrum, up and down the back at least x 3. Except for step 7a. above, this is the only procedure performed both up and down the back. All others are done up only, from sacrum to neck.

d.   <u>**Sound the High Jupiter 4th near the client's ears, circle around head, then move in a figure eight over the client, from crown to feet and back to the crown x 3.**</u>
The major energetic work of a Raindrop session has been done, and we relax for a few minutes to enjoy the bounty of it all.

STEP 8.   VALOR®.

a.   **Sprinkle Valor.** Sprinkle Valor oil directly on the spine with salt-shaker-like motion from sacrum to neck. Valor is a mild oil blend that does not get hot and can be applied generously.

b.   **3-6-12 Feathering Straight Up Spine.** Feather straight up spine as described STEP 4b. x 3.

c.   **Arched Feather Strokes (Angel Wings).** Feather with backs of fingernails in a curved fanning motion arched up and out to sides in 3" strokes (3x), 6" strokes (3x) and 12" strokes (3x).

d.   **Full Length Strokes.** Long feather strokes from sacrum up to and off of the shoulders as described in STEP 4e. 3x.

e.   <u>**Sound the High Saturn minor 2nd near the client's ears, circle around head, then move in a figure eight over the client, from crown to feet and back to the crown x 3.**</u>
We use this interval near the end of the Raindrop session to consolidate the endocrine and hormonal balancing that has begun with Raindrop.

STEP 9.   PEPPERMINT (use oil sparingly in this step, no more than 2-4 drops)

a.   **Raindrop Peppermint Oil.** Holding bottle of Peppermint about six inches above the client's back, drop only 2-3 drops directly on the spine from sacrum to neck.

b.   **3-6-12 Feathering Straight Up Spine.** Same procedure as Step 8b.

c.   **Arched Feather Strokes (Angel Wings).** Same procedure as Step 8c.

d.   **Full Length Strokes.** Same procedure as Step 8d.

STEP 10.   HOT COMPRESS.

a.   **Dry Towel.** Place large dry bath towel covering client's back from hips to atlas.

b.   **Hot Damp Towel.** Fold smaller towel into thirds, and roll into a cylinder. Then soak with hot water from the tap, wrung nearly dry, but still enough dampness to retain heat. Unroll the hot towel over the length of the spine from neck to hips.
* Multiple Sclerosis (MS). For people with MS, use a cold pack, NOT a hot pack. A towel soaked in cold water will do. An ice pack is also okay.

c.   **Another Dry Towel.** Lay another large towel over the compress to hold in heat.

d.   <u>**Sound the High Venus Minor 6th near the client's ears, circle around head, then move in a figure eight over the client, from crown to feet and back to the crown x 3.**</u>
Relax and know that the cleansing and release are perfect as the Venus energy brings the session to fullness.

e. <u>**Sound the Ohm Octave to the sole of each foot at KI 1 (Gushing Spring) x 3, right foot first.**</u>
The Ohm Octave brings feelings of comfort, completeness, and creates a sense of unity with All That Is. Thus ends our journey of healing with a Raindrop Technique session.

f. **Cooking the Client**. Oils will heat up and peak out in 5-8 minutes. If heat becomes too uncomfortable, apply V-6 or vegetable oil where needed. (See Note in Step 4.) Ask client to tell you when oils have cooled to a comfortable level.

g. **If Not Hot Enough**. If oils do not heat up with client, facilitator may place hands on back over the towel. NOTE: Because peppermint oil has been applied last, the client may experience what feels like coolness when, in fact, their back is warm.

STEP 11. REST & WATER

a. **Rest Quietly**. At this point client may wish to relax quietly for a few minutes. Whenever ready, they may sit up slowly with the facilitator standing nearby, being careful as they get off the massage table assisted by the facilitator.

b. **Drinking Water.** Have the client immediately drink a glass or bottle of good water and urge them to drink plenty of water for the next week.

STEP 12. RE-EVALUATION AND RE-MEASUREMENT.

a. **Measure Height Afterwards**. Re-measure client's height barefooted. Most will have grown from 1/4 to 1/2 inch. Those with severe spinal curvature may grow an inch or more. The benefits of Raindrop may not always include immediate growth but can be experienced by the receiver in other ways.

b. **Adjustments Continue for a Week.** A complete evaluation of the benefits received from Raindrop Technique may take several days to assess.

c. **Drink Lots of Water.** Remind the client to drink lots of water. The recommended amount is to divide their weight in pounds by two and drink that amount in ounces of pure (non-chlorinated) water every day.

---

* These notes correspond to a 120-min DVD entitled *Raindrop Technique*.
Available from CARE, RR 4 Box 646, Marble Hill, MO 63764
• (800) 758-8629 • or visit www.RaindropTraining.com.
Price: $29.95 + $9 s&h • Includes a set of notes

Additional Essential Oils Used
in Raindrop Technique for Joints & Bones

All of the Systems-specific Raindrop Technique protocol use Valor, oregano and thyme as the core three oils to open and close Raindrop Technique (EDOR, 4th Ed, page 299). Basil, marjoram, wintergreen, cypress and peppermint are replaced with oils more specific to the body system being treated. Details about the specific oils used to focus on the **Joints/Bones** system are included below.

HELICHRYSUM (*Helichrysum italicum*)--Family: Asteraceae (daisy); antispasmodic, detoxifier, regenerates nerves. Contains 28-60% esters, 16-22% ketones and 10-20% sesquiterpenes.

Cooling Helichrysum has an affinity for Lung and Liver meridians. It Clears Damp Heat Bi Obstruction and is excellent for breaking up fibrotic tissue. Can be very useful during a drug or chemical detox since it addresses Liver Fire leading to Liver Blood Stasis.

WINTERGREEN or **BIRCH** (**Gaultheria procumbens** or **Betula alleghaniensis**) - Family: Ericaceae (heather) or Family: Betulaceae (birch family) supports joints and skeletal structure. Composition of both of these oils are more than 80% methyl salicylate (a phenolic ester) which has a cortisone-like effect in that it may stimulate the body's own production of natural cortisone which has none of the untoward side-effects of synthetic cortisone. Also has analgesic properties inasmuch as its chemical structure is similar to that of aspirin.

Warming by nature and with an affinity for Bladder and Kidney meridians, Wintergreen expels Wind Damp Cold Bi Obstruction, so finds excellent application along the spine for chronic back problems.

SPRUCE (*Picea mariana*)--Family Pinaceae (pine); used for arthritis, rheumatism, sciatica, lumbago. Used by the Lakota to strengthen their ability to communicate with the Great Spirit. Traditionally believed to possess the frequency of prosperity. Contains 45-55% monoterpenes, 30-37% esters.

Spruce has an affinity for the Lung and Kidney meridians, and is warming. It is indicated for Deficient Kidney Yang and will expel wind Cold Bi Obstruction of back pain. Use for coughing and asthma to descend Lung Qi to the Kidneys.

PAN AWAY® (contains helichrysum, wintergreen, clove, and peppermint); reduces pain and inflammation, increases circulation and accelerates healing. Relieves swelling and pain from arthritis, sprains, muscle spasms and bruises.

PEPPERMINT (*Mentha piperita*) CT menthol - Family: Lamiaceae supports digestive system, respiratory system, and nervous system. Has been used for headaches. Research has shown that inhaling peppermint improves concentration and mental retention. Detoxing to the liver. A synergistic oil that supports and improves the beneficial actions of other oils used in conjunction. High in phenolics, but contains 9% sesquiterpenes.

Peppermint has an affinity for the Lung and Liver meridians with its cooling energy. Clears Wind Heat of headaches, fever, sore throat, and dry cough, as well as regulates Liver qi to promote menstruation, and decongest the Liver/PMS. It also promotes the movement of Wei qi.

Additional Intervals Used in Joint/Bone Raindrop Technique

Microtone - interval that is less than an equally spaced semitone, which in this case would be equal to 36.66 Hz in a twelve incremental Octave. The primary microtones in this system occur near the Unison, and are necessary to assist one to move away from grounding and center, to move away from a comfort zone in order to explore new possibilities and stimulate expansion and growth from within.

Mercury/Ohm - creates a great deal of movement and dissonance; volatile, going between the cracks, mental illumination and communication. Mercury has an affinity with the nervous system and communication of all kinds. Use this interval for all problems with the shoulders, arms and hands, especially if the nerves are involved.

Minor Second, 15:16

Mars/Ohm - harsh; carrier of considerable energetic potential, propels the mind, body and spirit into action with power and initiative to remove obstacles. This interval is used all muscle problems such as atrophy, hypertrophy, spasm, and influences the proper functioning of the muscle system. This interval is also used near the end of the journey, when we need to mobilize our energies and courage to move and release the unnecessary burdens that we carry.

Saturn/Ohm - semitone and somewhat dissonant, supports the formation of new boundaries and structures. The Minor Second is the most dissonant of the intervals, and Saturn/Ohm is more dissonant than Mars/Ohm. They both represent the applications of energy toward the manifestation of material form, in other words creating matter from spirit. Twin pillars of evolution on the material and spiritual planes. Use this interval for all problems with skeleton, arthritis, chronic subluxations, cartilage, ligaments and fascia.

JOINTS & BONES
Vibrational Raindrop

Based on Raindrop Technique as Taught by D. Gary Young
At the Young Living Level I Training Conference in
Dallas, Texas, January 25-29, 2000
(From the CARE Raindrop Training Notes)

**The notes in Underlined Helvetica Bold are the tuning fork applications
to be done with the Joint/Bone Raindrop Tuning Kit**

• **NOTE:**   The person receiving oils is called the "client" or the "receiver." The person administering the oils is called the "facilitator." While this is the version of Raindrop taught by CARE Instructors, you may adapt the tuning forks to be used after the appropriate oils in different versions of Raindrop.

• **PRELIMINARIES:** Facilitator should trim nails as short as possible and file sharp corners and edges. Facilitator and client should both remove all metal, especially rings, bracelets, and watches.

STEP 1.   EVALUATION, PREPARATION AND PERMISSION.

a.   **Measure Height** of the client barefooted using a square box against a wall and sliding down to the head to assure a level measurement. This is not an essential part of raindrop, but is an objective demonstration of what often happens. Most people grow a little with a raindrop, but if one does not grow, that does not mean the raindrop has been ineffective or erroneously per formed.

b.   **Allergies, Sensitivities, Toxicity, etc.** Ask if client is prone to allergies, reactions to drugs or has developed any sensitizations to any sub stances. Mention to the client that allergic reactions to therapeutic grade essential oils are not possible, but sometimes there can be a detox reaction. Ask if they smoke or if they have ever engaged in occu pations exposing them to chemicals such as beauty shop, auto body, professional housecleaning, pesticides, herbicides, photo chemicals, environmental engineering, hospitals, etc.

c.   **Suggested Resources with Cleansing Information**: *Essential Oils Desk Reference*; *Reference Guide for Essential Oils*; *Healing for the Age of Enlightenment*.

d.   **Ask Permission.** After explaining the procedure to the client, ask per mission to continue.

e.   **Bathroom:** Ask if client needs to use bathroom before you start.

f.   **Bodily Contact:** Once session begins, the facilitator should try to keep bodily contact with client at all times. When tuning forks are sound ed around the client, the facilitator will need to break bodily contact to do this technique.

• HAVE CLIENT LIE FACE UP

STEP 2. VALOR®.
a. **Listen to the Ohm Unison x 3 (hold tuning forks to client's ears).**
b. **Shoulders.** Place 3 drops of Valor on each shoulder. Hold for 5 minutes or more until a balance of energies is felt. Place your left hand on the left shoulder and your right hand on the right shoulder.
c. **Soles of Feet.** Place 6 drops of Valor on the soles of each foot. Cross your arms so your right hand holds the right foot and your left hand holds the left foot. You will have to cross your arms to accomplish this.
d. **Sound the Ohm Unison to the sole of each foot at KI 1 (Gushing Spring) and at KI 3 (Great Ravine) in the depression behind the inner ankle x 3, right foot first.** We begin the Raindrop journey from a firm, grounded place within. This interval deeply roots our core essence.

STEP 3. VALOR, OREGANO, THYME, HELICHRYSUM, WINTERGREEN, PANAWAY, SPRUCE and PEPPERMINT.
a. **Foot Vita Flex.** Vita Flex on each foot along spinal reflex points, coccyx to brain, starting with right foot. Each foot should be done with 2-3 drops per foot of each of the 8 oils in the order listed x 3.
b. **Sound the Ohm Octave with Low Ohm at CV4 (Origin Pass) on the abdomen four finger-widths below the umbilicus, and Ohm at CV17 (Chest Center) in the center of the chest level with the 4th rib, x 3.**
This interval creates a harmonic bridge and connection between the upper and lower body, further rooting our core energy.

• HAVE CLIENT ROLL OVER TO A FACE DOWN POSITION

STEP 4. DUO: OREGANO AND THYME.*
a. **Raindrop Oregano.** Holding bottle of Oregano about six inches above the client's back, drop 4-6 drops directly on the spine from sacrum to neck.
b. **3-6-12 Feathering Straight Up Spine.** Feather stroke Oregano straight up the spine with a light touch using backs of fingernails gently brushing against client's skin. Start with 3" strokes alternately with each hand x 3 the length of the spine upwards to the atlas vertebra, then 6" strokes x 3, followed by 12" strokes x 3.
c. **Thyme Raindrop.** Repeat a. & b. above for Thyme.
d. **Feathering Straight to Sides.** After both Oregano and Thyme have been applied, starting at the sacrum, feather oils away from spine straight out nd down the sides x 3, then move up half-a-hand's width and repeat until you reach the neck and skull. Repeat this sacrum to atlas x 3.
e. **Full Length Strokes.** Long feather strokes, both hands side by side, touching with back of nail tips only along both sides of the spine, sweep full length from sacrum to base of neck, fanning out and off the shoulders x 3.

71

f. **Sound the Solar 7th with the Low Ohm on GV2 (Low Back Shu) at base of sacrum and Sun fork on GV16 (Wind Mansion) on the back of the skull one inch above the posterior hairline.**

This interval assists the core Duo of Oregano and Thyme to "heat up" the cells and cleanse them for deletion of old, redundant and useless information. These two points achieve "cranial-sacral stillpoint" from which changes can occur and a new order can be achieved.

* Important Note. Some oils (particularly Oregano and Thyme) can cause heat when in contact with the skin and react with viruses, bacteria, and toxins. This is generally a good sign that the oils are seeking out and destroying harmful aliens that hibernate in the fatty tissue and lymph nodes along the spine. However, if at any time the heat becomes unpleasant for the client, apply V-6 or other vegetable oil where indicated. Relief should be immediate. Ask the client to tell you when and where this is needed throughout the Raindrop Technique session

STEP 5. TRIO: HELICHRYSUM, WINTERGREEN AND PANAWAY

a. **Raindrop the Oils on the Back in the Order Given**. Follow steps a. & b. of STEP 4 above with Helichrysum, Wintergreen and Panaway instead of Oregano and Thyme.

b. **Finger Circles.** After all three oils have been applied, apply your fingers to the laminar groove along one side of the spine, slowly progressing from sacrum to atlas, using four fingers of both hands together in a clockwise motion, pulling tissues away from spine with each circle. Then walk around table and go up other side. Alternate from side to side, right to left, until both sides have been done x 3. Apply Aroma Seiz® where tense muscles are discovered.

c. **Sound Zodiac 3rd wherever muscle knots are found at least x 3 at each location.**

If it is too painful to use the forks at the same location, then one fork can be placed on either side of the location of spasm.

*Note on Additional Oils: At this point, before the finger circles, additional oils (such as Joy®, Frankincense, Release®, Relieve It®, Harmony®, Panaway®, etc.) may be applied if desired according to the wishes, needs, or special circumstances of the client. With each additional oil, drop them raindrop-style directly on the spine and then stroke them straight up the spine with the 3-6-12 feathering described in STEPS 4a and 4b. described above. **If other oils are added, sound the High Full Moon 6th near the client's ears, circle around head, then move in a figure eight over the client, from crown to feet and back to the crown x 3.** Relax and know that the cleansing and release are perfect and enjoy a sense of magic and fulfillment, with a pull towards healing that allows one's potential to manifest.*

STEP 6.   SPRUCE.

a.   **Sprinkle Spruce.** Sprinkle Spruce oil directly on the spine with a salt-shaker-like motion from sacrum to neck.

b.   **3-6-12 Feathering Straight Up Spine.** Feather straight up spine as described in STEP 4b. x 3.

c.   **Thumb Vita Flex.** Thumb Vita Flex along sides of spine from sacrum to atlas x 3.

d.   **Saw Maneuver & Skull-Pull.** Apply saw maneuver from sacrum to neck with three skull-pulls x 3.

e.   **Spine Stretch & Shake (or Quiver).** Apply two-handed spine stretch maneuver vibrating with a shaking or quivering motion perpendicular to the spine with each stretch, moving gradually upwards from sacrum to atlas. 3x.

f.   **Sound the appropriate interval around the joint/area in question: Use the Mercury Microtone for the shoulders, the Saturn Minor 2nd for the knees, and the Mars Minor 2nd for general muscle pain.**
Use the Mercury Microtone interval for all problems with the shoulders, arms and hands, especially if the nerves are involved. Use the Saturn Minor 2nd interval for all problems with skeleton, arthritis, chronic subluxations, cartilage, ligaments and fascia. Use the Mars Minor 2nd interval for all muscle problems such as atrophy, hypertrophy, spasm, and influences the proper functioning of the muscle system.

STEP 7.   ORTHO EASE®.

a.   **Apply Ortho Ease Oil.** Dispense oil generously onto palms first, then apply over the entire back, spreading it with flat palms of the hands in clockwise circular movements from hips to neck, cross over, and then back down to the hips. Repeat x 3. A free style anointing without structure or counting may be done. Include attention of the shoulder blades, neck, trapezium muscles, and places that are tight or sore. Ask client if they have any particular requests in this regard.

b.   **(Optional) Rest** Quietly rest face down for 4-5 minutes. Cover with sheet to keep client warm and comfortable, if necessary. Apply more Ortho Ease as needed, repeating step 7a.

c.   **Indian Rub.** Perform see-saw rub maneuver across the spine progressing from sacrum to neck and from neck to sacrum, up and down the back at least x 3. Except for step 7a. above, this is the only procedure performed both up and down the back. All others are done up only, from sacrum to neck.

d.   **Sound the High Jupiter 4th near the client's ears, circle around head, then move in a figure eight over the client, from crown to feet and back to the crown x 3.**
The major energetic work of a Raindrop session has been done, and we can relax for a few minutes to enjoy the bounty of it all.

STEP 8.   VALOR®.

a.   **Sprinkle Valor.** Sprinkle Valor oil directly on the spine with salt-shaker-like motion from sacrum to neck. Valor is a mild oil blend that does not get hot and can be applied generously.

b.   **3-6-12 Feathering Straight Up Spine.** Feather straight up spine as described STEP 4b. x 3.

c.   **Arched Feather Strokes (Angel Wings).** Feather with backs of fingernails in a curved fanning motion arched up and out to sides in 3" strokes (3x), 6" strokes (3x) and 12" strokes (3x).

d.   **Full Length Strokes.** Long feather strokes from sacrum up to and off of the shoulders as described in STEP 4e. 3x.

e.   <u>**Sound the High Mars minor 2nd near the client's ears, circle around head, then move in a figure eight over the client, from crown to feet and back to the crown x 3.**</u>
We are near the end of the journey, and need to mobilize our energies and courage to expel the unnecessary burdens which we carry. Mars is associated with the adrenals and perfectly suited to resolve the imbalances associated with chronic stress.

STEP 9.   PEPPERMINT (use oil sparingly in this step, no more than 2-4 drops)

a.   **Raindrop Peppermint Oil.** Holding bottle of Peppermint about six inches above the client's back, drop only 2-3 drops directly on the spine from sacrum to neck.

b.   **3-6-12 Feathering Straight Up Spine.** Same procedure as Step 8b.

c.   **Arched Feather Strokes (Angel Wings).** Same procedure as Step 8c.

d.   **Full Length Strokes.** Same procedure as Step 8d.

STEP 10. HOT COMPRESS.

a.   **Dry Towel.** Place large dry bath towel covering client's back from hips to atlas.

b.   **Hot Damp Towel.** Fold smaller towel into thirds, and roll into a cylinder. Then soak with hot water from the tap, wrung nearly dry, but still enough dampness to retain heat. Unroll the hot towel over the length of the spine from neck to hips.
    * **Multiple Sclerosis (MS).** For people with MS, use a cold pack, NOT a hot pack. A towel soaked in cold water will do. An ice pack is also okay.

c.   **Another Dry Towel.** Lay another large towel over the compress to hold in heat.

d.   <u>**Sound the Full Moon Major 6th near the client's ears, circle around head, then move in a figure eight over the client, from crown to feet and back to the crown x 3.**</u>
Relax and know that the cleansing and release are perfect as the Venus energy brings the session to fullness.

e. **Sound the Ohm Octave to the sole of each foot at KI 1 (Gushing Spring) x 3, right foot first.**
    The Ohm Octave brings feelings of comfort, completeness, and creates a sense of unity with All That Is. Thus ends our journey of healing with a Raindrop Technique session.

f. **Cooking the Client**. Oils will heat up and peak out in 5-8 minutes. If heat becomes too uncomfortable, apply V-6 or vegetable oil where needed. (See Note in Step 4.) Ask client to tell you when oils have cooled to a comfortable level.

g. **If Not Hot Enough**. If oils do not heat up with client, facilitator may place hands on back over the towel. NOTE: Because peppermint oil has been applied last, the client may experience what feels like coolness when, in fact, their back is warm.

STEP 11. REST & WATER
a. **Rest Quietly**. At this point client may wish to relax quietly for a few minutes. Whenever ready, they may sit up slowly with the facilitator standing nearby, being careful as they get off the massage table assisted by the facilitator.

b. **Drinking Water.** Have the client immediately drink a glass or bottle of good water and urge them to drink plenty of water for the next week.

STEP 12. RE-EVALUATION AND RE-MEASUREMENT.
a. **Measure Height Afterwards**. Re-measure client's height barefooted. Most will have grown from 1/4 to 1/2 inch. Those with severe spinal curvature may grow an inch or more. The benefits of Raindrop may not always include immediate growth but can be experienced by the receiver in other ways.

b. **Adjustments Continue for a Week.** A complete evaluation of the benefits received from Raindrop Technique may take several days to assess.

c. **Drink Lots of Water.** Remind the client to drink lots of water. The recommended amount is to divide their weight in pounds by two and drink that amount in ounces of pure (non-chlorinated) water every day.

---

* These notes correspond to a 120-min DVD entitled *Raindrop Technique*.
Available from CARE, RR 4 Box 646, Marble Hill, MO 63764
• (800) 758-8629 • or visit www.RaindropTraining.com.
Price: $29.95 + $9 s&h • Includes a set of notes

Additional Essential Oils
Used in Raindrop Technique for Liver

All of the Systems-specific Raindrop Technique protocol use Valor, oregano and thyme as the core three oils to open and close Raindrop Technique (EDOR, 4th Ed, page 299). Basil, marjoram, wintergreen, cypress and peppermint are replaced with oils more specific to the body system being treated. Details about the specific oils used to focus on the **Liver** system are included below.

JUVAFLEX® (contains geranium, rosemary, Roman Chamomile, fennel, helichrysum and blue tansy); supports liver and lymphatic detoxification, helps break addictions to coffee, drugs, alcohol, tobacco and anger.

GERMAN CHAMOMILE (*Matricaria recutita*)--Family: Asteraceae (daisy); powerful antioxidant (inhibits lipid perosidation), anti-inflammatory, promotes digestion, liver and gallbladder health. Dispels anger, helps release emotions linked to the past. Soothes and clears the mind. Contains 33-57% oxides, 34-60% sesquiterpenes.

Cooling and with an affinity for the Liver and Heart meridians, German Chamomile clears Liver Fire and subdues Liver Wind to assist with headaches, anger outbursts, diaphragmatic construction and muscle cramps. It calms the Shen to reduce anxiety. German Chamomile also harmonizes Liver and its effect on the Stomach with symptoms of IBS, candida, and ulcers.

CARROT SEED (*Daucus carota*)--Family Apiacea (parsley family); traditionally used for kidney and digestive disorders and to relieve liver congestion, water retention. Contains 29-47% alcohols, 20-24% monoterpenes, 14-18% sesquiterpenes.

Cooling Carrot Seed nourishes Liver Blood and has an affinity for the Liver and Kidney meridians. It is indicated for Deficient Liver Blood symptoms of dry eyes, poor vision, dizziness and brittle nails. Carrot Seed oil can also regulate the production of thyroxine.

LEDUM (*Ledum groenlandicum*)--Family: Ericaceae (heather family); diuretic, liver-protectant, used for liver problems, hepatitis, fatty liver, obesity and water retention. Contains 30-50% monoterpenes, 13-20% sesquiterpenes.

Cooling in nature, Ledum has an affinity for the Liver and Spleen meridians. Use it for Liver Qi Stagnation to promote the smooth flow of Liver qi and resolve headaches, abdominal pain, and muscle spasms. Also indicated to Calm the Shen and resolves symptoms of irritability, restlessness and high blood pressure (Liver Fire).

PEPPERMINT (*Mentha piperita*) CT menthol - Family: Lamiaceae supports digestive system, respiratory system, and nervous system. Has been used for headaches. Research has shown that inhaling peppermint improves concentration and mental retention. Detoxing to the liver. A synergistic oil that supports and improves the beneficial actions of other oils used in conjunction. High in phenolics, but contains 9% sesquiterpenes.

Peppermint has an affinity for the Lung and Liver meridians with its cooling energy. Clears Wind Heat of headaches, fever, sore throat, and dry cough, as well as regulates Liver qi to promote menstruation, and decongest the Liver/PMS. It also promotes the movement of Wei qi.

Additional Intervals
Used in Liver Raindrop Technique

Microtone - interval that is less than an equally spaced semitone, which in this case would be equal to 36.66 Hz in a twelve incremental Octave. The primary microtones in this system occur near the Unison, and are necessary to assist one to move away from grounding and center, to move away from a comfort zone in order to explore new possibilities and stimulate expansion and growth from within.

High Pluto/High Ohm - highly dissonant, penetrates deep into the body structure to a cellular level, breaks down resistance to change, unconscious and shadow self level. Disharmony between notes creates desire for resolution. As the Liver is cleansed, toxins can manifest on the skin; this interval helps to bring the toxins to the surface and clear them.

Major Third, 4:5
High Zodiac Earth/High Ohm - optimistic, happy; meditative, dispersive or dispelling effect, relieves mental stress, but is especially useful to relieve physical stress. We use this interval to release stagnant Liver energy, which can be seen in problems such as hot flashes, PMS symptoms, headaches, and anger/frustration issues.

Fourth, 3:4
Jupiter/Ohm - Perfect Fourth; pure, like church bells; stimulates growth, abundance and expansion. The Fourth is the geometric mean of an Octave. Jupiter has a natural affinity for the Liver which allows it to influence the production of bile, cholesterol, and glycogen production. Jupiter is also associated with the sciatic nerve, the hips and thighs.

LIVER
Vibrational Raindrop

Based on Raindrop Technique as Taught by D. Gary Young
At the Young Living Level I Training Conference in
Dallas, Texas, January 25-29, 2000
(From the CARE Raindrop Training Notes)

The notes in Underlined Helvetica Bold are the tuning fork applications
to be done with the Liver Raindrop Tuning Kit

• **NOTE:** The person receiving oils is called the "client" or the "receiver." The person administering the oils is called the "facilitator." While this is the version of Raindrop taught by CARE Instructors, you may adapt the tuning forks to be used after the appropriate oils in different versions of Raindrop.

• **PRELIMINARIES:** Facilitator should trim nails as short as possible and file sharp corners and edges. Facilitator and client should both remove all metal, especially rings, bracelets, and watches.

STEP 1. EVALUATION, PREPARATION AND PERMISSION.
a. **Measure Height** of the client barefooted using a square box against a wall and sliding down to the head to assure a level measurement. This is not an essential part of raindrop, but is an objective demonstration of what often happens. Most people grow a little with a raindrop, but if one does not grow, that does not mean the raindrop has been ineffective or erroneously per formed.
b. **Allergies, Sensitivities, Toxicity, etc.** Ask if client is prone to allergies, reactions to drugs or has developed any sensitizations to any sub stances. Mention to the client that allergic reactions to therapeutic grade essential oils are not possible, but sometimes there can be a detox reaction. Ask if they smoke or if they have ever engaged in occu pations exposing them to chemicals such as beauty shop, auto body, professional housecleaning, pesticides, herbicides, photo chemicals, environmental engineering, hospitals, etc.
c. **Suggested Resources with Cleansing Information**: *Essential Oils Desk Reference*; *Reference Guide for Essential Oils*; *Healing for the Age of Enlightenment*.
d. **Ask Permission.** After explaining the procedure to the client, ask per mission to continue.
e. **Bathroom:** Ask if client needs to use bathroom before you start.
f. **Bodily Contact:** Once session begins, the facilitator should try to keep bodily contact with client at all times. When tuning forks are sounded around the client, the facilitator will need to break bodily contact to do this technique.

LIVER

• **HAVE CLIENT LIE FACE UP**

STEP 2.   VALOR®.

a.   <u>**Listen to the Ohm Unison x 3 (hold tuning forks to client's ears).**</u>

b.   **Shoulders.** Place 3 drops of Valor on each shoulder. Hold for 5 minutes or more until a balance of energies is felt. Place your left hand on the left shoulder and your right hand on the right shoulder.

c.   **Soles of Feet.** Place 6 drops of Valor on the soles of each foot. Cross your arms so your right hand holds the right foot and your left hand holds the left foot. You will have to cross your arms to accomplish this.

d.   <u>**Sound the Ohm Unison to the sole of each foot at KI 1 (Gushing Spring) and at KI 3 (Great Ravine) in the depression behind the inner ankle x 3, right foot first.**</u> We begin the Raindrop journey from a firm, grounded place within. This interval deeply roots our core essence.

STEP 3.   VALOR, OREGANO, THYME, CARROT SEED,
**   GERMAN CHAMOMILE, JUVAFLEX, LEDUM and PEPPERMINT.**

a.   **Foot Vita Flex.** Vita Flex on each foot along spinal reflex points, coccyx to brain, starting with right foot. Each foot should be done with 2-3 drops per foot of each of the 8 oils in the order listed x 3.

b.   <u>**Sound the Ohm Octave with Low Ohm at CV4 (Origin Pass) on the abdomen four finger-widths below the umbilicus, and Ohm at CV17 (Chest Center) in the center of the chest level with the 4th rib, x 3.**</u>
         This interval creates a harmonic bridge and connection between the upper and lower body, further rooting our core energy.

• **HAVE CLIENT ROLL OVER TO A FACE DOWN POSITION**

STEP 4.   DUO: OREGANO AND THYME.*

a.   **Raindrop Oregano.** Holding bottle of Oregano about six inches above the client's back, drop 4-6 drops directly on the spine from sacrum to neck.

b.   **3-6-12 Feathering Straight Up Spine.** Feather stroke Oregano straight up the spine with a light touch using backs of fingernails gently brushing against client's skin. Start with 3" strokes alternately with each hand x 3 the length of the spine upwards to the atlas vertebra, then 6" strokes x 3, followed by 12" strokes x 3.

c.   **Thyme Raindrop.** Repeat a. & b. above for Thyme.

d.   **Feathering Straight to Sides.** After both Oregano and Thyme have been applied, starting at the sacrum, feather oils away from spine straight out nd down the sides x 3, then move up half-a-hand's width and repeat until you reach the neck and skull. Repeat this sacrum to atlas x 3.

e.   **Full Length Strokes.** Long feather strokes, both hands side by side, touching with back of nail tips only along both sides of the spine, sweep full length from sacrum to base of neck, fanning out and off the shoulders x 3.

f. <u>**Sound the Solar 7th with the Low Ohm on GV2 (Low Back Shu) at base of sacrum and Sun fork on GV16 (Wind Mansion) on the back of the skull one inch above the posterior hairline.**</u>
This interval assists the core Duo of Oregano and Thyme to "heat up" the cells and cleanse them for deletion of old, redundant and useless information. These two points achieve "cranial-sacral stillpoint" from which changes can occur and a new order can be achieved.

* Important Note. *Some oils (particularly Oregano and Thyme) can cause heat when in contact with the skin and react with viruses, bacteria, and toxins. This is generally a good sign that the oils are seeking out and destroying harmful aliens that hibernate in the fatty tissue and lymph nodes along the spine. However, if at any time the heat becomes unpleasant for the client, apply V-6 or other vegetable oil where indicated. Relief should be immediate. Ask the client to tell you when and where this is needed throughout the Raindrop Technique session*

STEP 5.   TRIO: CARROT SEED, GERMAN CHAMOMILE AND JUVAFLEX

a. **Raindrop the Oils on the Back in the Order Given**. Follow steps a. & b. of STEP 4 above with Carrot Seed, German Chamomile and Juvaflex instead of Oregano and Thyme.

b. **Finger Circles**. After all three oils have been applied, apply your fingers to the laminar groove along one side of the spine, slowly progressing from sacrum to atlas, using four fingers of both hands together in a clockwise motion, pulling tissues away from spine with each circle. Then walk around table and go up other side. Alternate from side to side, right to left, until both sides have been done x 3. Apply AromaSiez® where tense muscles are discovered.

c. <u>**Sound Zodiac 3rd wherever muscle knots are found at least x 3 at each location.**</u> If it is too painful to use the forks at the same location, then one fork can be placed on either side of the location of spasm.

Note on Additional Oils: *At this point, before the finger circles, additional oils (such as Joy®, Frankincense, Release®, Relieve It®, Harmony®, Panaway®, etc.) may be applied if desired according to the wishes, needs, or special circumstances of the client. With each additional oil, drop them raindrop-style directly on the spine and then stroke them straight up the spine with the 3-6-12 feathering described in STEPS 4a and 4b. described above.* <u>**If other oils are added, sound the High Full Moon 6th near the client's ears, circle around head, then move in a figure eight over the client, from crown to feet and back to the crown x 3.**</u> *Relax and know that the cleansing and release are perfect and enjoy a sense of magic and fulfillment, with a pull towards healing that allows one's potential to manifest.*

STEP 6.   LEDUM.

a.   **Sprinkle Ledum**. Sprinkle Ledum oil directly on the spine with a salt-shaker-like motion from sacrum to neck.

b.   **3-6-12 Feathering Straight Up Spine**. Feather straight up spine as described in STEP 4b. x 3.

c.   **Thumb Vita Flex.** Thumb Vita Flex along sides of spine from sacrum to atlas x 3.

d.   **Saw Maneuver & Skull-Pull.** Apply saw maneuver from sacrum to neck with three skull-pulls x 3.

e.   **Spine Stretch & Shake (or Quiver)**. Apply two-handed spine stretch maneuver vibrating with a shaking or quivering motion perpendicular to the spine with each stretch, moving gradually upwards from sacrum to atlas. 3x.

f.   <u>**Sound the Jupiter 4th on the Huato Jiaji points up the spine from sacrum to base of skull. The Huato Jiaji points are found on either side of the spine between the vertebrae. Then hold both forks together at GV20 (Hundred Convergences) in the depression at the crown of the head and also near he ears to allow client to hear the interval.**</u>
Jupiter has a natural affinity for the Liver which allows it to influence the production of bile, cholesterol, and glycogen production. Jupiter is also associated with the sciatic nerve, the hips and thighs.

STEP 7.   ORTHO EASE®.

a.   **Apply Ortho Ease Oil**. Dispense oil generously onto palms first, then apply over the entire back, spreading it with flat palms of the hands in clockwise circular movements from hips to neck, cross over, and then back down to the hips. Repeat x 3. A free style anointing without structure or counting may be done. Include attention of the shoulder blades, neck, trapezium muscles, and places that are tight or sore. Ask client if they have any particular requests in this regard.

b.   **(Optional) Rest** Quietly rest face down for 4-5 minutes. Cover with sheet to keep client warm and comfortable, if necessary. Apply more Ortho Ease as needed, repeating step 7a.

c.   **Indian Rub.** Perform see-saw rub maneuver across the spine progressing from sacrum to neck and from neck to sacrum, up and down the back at least x 3. Except for step 7a. above, this is the only procedure performed both up and down the back. All others are done up only, from sacrum to neck.

d.   <u>**Sound the High Zodiac 3rd near the client's ears, circle around head, then move in a figure eight over the client, from crown to feet and back to the crown x 3.**</u>
We use this interval to release stagnant Liver energy, which can be seen in problems such as hot flashes, PMS symptoms, headaches, and anger/frustration issues.

STEP 8.   VALOR®.

a.   **Sprinkle Valor.** Sprinkle Valor oil directly on the spine with salt-shaker-
     like motion from sacrum to neck. Valor is a mild oil blend that does not
     get hot and can be applied generously.

b.   **3-6-12 Feathering Straight Up Spine**. Feather straight up spine as
     described STEP 4b. x 3.

c.   **Arched Feather Strokes (Angel Wings)**. Feather with backs of fingernails
     in a curved fanning motion arched up and out to sides in 3" strokes (3x),
     6" strokes (3x) and 12" strokes (3x).

d.   **Full Length Strokes.** Long feather strokes from sacrum up to and off of
     the shoulders as described in STEP 4e. 3x.

e.   <u>**Sound the High Pluto Microtone near the client's ears, circle around head,
     then move in a figure eight over the client, from crown to feet and back to
     the crown x 3.**</u>
     As the Liver is cleansed, toxins can manifest on the skin; this interval
     helps to bring the toxins to the surface and clear them.

**STEP 9.   PEPPERMINT (use oil sparingly in this step, no more than
             2-4 drops)**

a.   **Raindrop Peppermint Oil.** Holding bottle of Peppermint about six
     inches above the client's back, drop only 2-3 drops directly on the spine
     from sacrum to neck.

b.   **3-6-12 Feathering Straight Up Spine.** Same procedure as Step 8b.

c.   **Arched Feather Strokes (Angel Wings)**. Same procedure as Step 8c.

d.   **Full Length Strokes**. Same procedure as Step 8d.

STEP 10. HOT COMPRESS.

a.   **Dry Towel.** Place large dry bath towel covering client's back from hips
     to atlas.

b.   **Hot Damp Towel**. Fold smaller towel into thirds, and roll into a cylinder.
     Then soak with hot water from the tap, wrung nearly dry, but still enough
     dampness to retain heat. Unroll the hot towel over the length of the spine
     from neck to hips.
     * Multiple Sclerosis (MS). For people with MS, use a cold pack, NOT a
     hot pack. A towel soaked in cold water will do. An ice pack is also okay.

c.   **Another Dry Towel.** Lay another large towel over the compress to hold
     in heat.

d.   <u>**Sound the Zodiac Earth Major 3rd near the client's ears, circle around head,
     then move in a figure eight over the client, from crown to feet and back to
     the crown x 3.**</u>
     Relax and know that the cleansing and release are perfect as the
     Venus energy brings the session to fullness.

e. <u>**Sound the Ohm Octave to the sole of each foot at KI 1 (Gushing Spring) x 3,**</u>
<u>**right foot first.**</u>
The Ohm Octave brings feelings of comfort, completeness, and creates a
sense of unity with All That Is. Thus ends our journey of healing with a
Raindrop Technique session.

f. **Cooking the Client**. Oils will heat up and peak out in 5-8 minutes. If
heat becomes too uncomfortable, apply V-6 or vegetable oil where needed.
(See Note in Step 4.) Ask client to tell you when oils have cooled to a
comfortable level.

g. **If Not Hot Enough**. If oils do not heat up with client, facilitator may place
hands on back over the towel. NOTE: Because peppermint oil has been
applied last, the client may experience what feels like coolness when, in
fact, their back is warm.

STEP 11. REST & WATER

a. **Rest Quietly**. At this point client may wish to relax quietly for a few
minutes. Whenever ready, they may sit up slowly with the facilitator
standing nearby, being careful as they get off the massage table assisted
by the facilitator.

b. **Drinking Water.** Have the client immediately drink a glass or bottle of
good water and urge them to drink plenty of water for the next week.

STEP 12. RE-EVALUATION AND RE-MEASUREMENT.

a. **Measure Height Afterwards**. Re-measure client's height barefooted.
Most will have grown from 1/4 to 1/2 inch. Those with severe spinal
curvature may grow an inch or more. The benefits of Raindrop may not
always include immediate growth but can be experienced by the receiver
in other ways.

b. **Adjustments Continue for a Week.** A complete evaluation of the benefits
received from Raindrop Technique may take several days to assess.

c. **Drink Lots of Water.** Remind the client to drink lots of water. The recommended amount is to divide their weight in pounds by two and drink that
amount in ounces of pure (non-chlorinated) water every day.

---

* These notes correspond to a 120-min DVD entitled *Raindrop Technique*.
Available from CARE, RR 4 Box 646, Marble Hill, MO 63764
• (800) 758-8629 • or visit <u>www.RaindropTraining.com</u>.
Price: $29.95 + $9 s&h • Includes a set of notes

Additional Essential Oils
Used in Lung Raindrop Technique

All of the Systems-specific Raindrop Technique protocol use Valor, oregano and thyme as the core three oils to open and close Raindrop Technique (EDOR, 4th Ed, page 299). Basil, marjoram, wintergreen, cypress and peppermint are replaced with oils more specific to the body system being treated. Details about the specific oils used to focus on the **Lung** system are included below.

RAVENSARA (*Ravensara aromatica*)--Family: Lamiaceae (mint family); antimicrobial and supporting to the nerves and respiratory system, called "the oil that heals" by the people of Madagascar. Contains 48-61% oxides, 16-32% monoterpenes.

Ravensara is neutral and has an affinity to the Lung and Liver meridians. It can be used to Clear Wind Heat and Lung Heat with symptoms of fever, cough and wheezing. It can also be used for Lung Wind Cold with chest congestion and pain. Very pungent and dispersing, strongly anti-viral essential oil.

MELROSE® (contains melaleuca, naouli, rosemary and clove); a strong topical antiseptic that cleans and disinfects cuts, scrapes, burns, rashes and bruised tissue. Helps regenerate damaged tissue and reduce inflammation.

EUCALYPTUS RADIATA (*Eucalyptus radiata*)--Family: Myrtaceae (myrtle); antibacterial, antiviral, expectorant, used in respiratory and sinus infections; fights Herpes simplex when combined with bergamot. Contains 61-77% oxides, 13-24% monoterpenes.

Warming with an affinity to the Lung and Stomach meridians, Eucalyptus Radiata is useful to treat Wind Cold with chills and fever, body aches, headaches and pain. It can be applied directly to the chest for Hot Phlegm and will expel Damp Phlegm.

MYRTLE (*Myrtus communis*)--Family: Myrtaceae (myrtle); normalizes hormonal imbalances, thyroid problems, prostate problems, muscle spasms. Contains 31-48% oxides, 30-45% monoterpenes.

Dry and cool, Myrtle clears Lung Heat and astringes leakage of qi and Blood such as sweating, bleeding, diarrhea and hemorrhoids. It is calming as a nervine.

RAVEN® (contains ravensara, eucalyptus radiata, peppermint, wintergreen, and lemon); treats respiratory disease and infections such as tuberculosis, influenza and pneumonia; highly antiviral and antiseptic.

Additional Intervals
Used in Lung Raindrop Technique

Major Sixth, 3:5

Full Moon/Ohm - Optimistic, less emotional than the Major 3rd; builds energy, brings a feeling of fellness, unveiling, and purification; the ultimate expression of Yin. Can bring a sense of magic and fulfillment; is rhythmic with a pull towards healing that allows one's potential to manifest. Known as the Golden Section, Divine Proportion, or Golden Mean. This interval builds yin energy, which moistens, consolidates and cools the body. It is especially effective for lung dryness that may come from smoking or emphysema.

Fifth, 2:3

High New Moon/High Ohm - calming, relaxing, opening. The New Moon 5th is dispersive for emotional issues, while the Earth Day 5th is better suited to gather and strengthen energy. This intervals opens, releases and dispels the stagnant energy that has accumulated during the Raindrop session, and is especially useful for asthma and lung congestion.

LUNG
Vibrational Raindrop

Based on Raindrop Technique as Taught by D. Gary Young
At the Young Living Level I Training Conference in
Dallas, Texas, January 25-29, 2000
(From the CARE Raindrop Training Notes)

The notes in Underlined Helvetica Bold are the tuning fork applications to be done with the Lung Raindrop Tuning Kit

• **NOTE:** The person receiving oils is called the "client" or the "receiver." The person administering the oils is called the "facilitator." While this is the version of Raindrop taught by CARE Instructors, you may adapt the tuning forks to be used after the appropriate oils in different versions of Raindrop.

• **PRELIMINARIES:** Facilitator should trim nails as short as possible and file sharp corners and edges. Facilitator and client should both remove all metal, especially rings, bracelets, and watches.

STEP 1. EVALUATION, PREPARATION AND PERMISSION.

a. **Measure Height** of the client barefooted using a square box against a wall and sliding down to the head to assure a level measurement. This is not an essential part of raindrop, but is an objective demonstration of what often happens. Most people grow a little with a raindrop, but if one does not grow, that does not mean the raindrop has been ineffective or erroneously per formed.

b. **Allergies, Sensitivities, Toxicity, etc.** Ask if client is prone to allergies, reactions to drugs or has developed any sensitizations to any sub stances. Mention to the client that allergic reactions to therapeutic grade essential oils are not possible, but sometimes there can be a detox reaction. Ask if they smoke or if they have ever engaged in occu pations exposing them to chemicals such as beauty shop, auto body, professional housecleaning, pesticides, herbicides, photo chemicals, environmental engineering, hospitals, etc.

c. **Suggested Resources with Cleansing Information:** *Essential Oils Desk Reference; Reference Guide for Essential Oils; Healing for the Age of Enlightenment.*

d. **Ask Permission.** After explaining the procedure to the client, ask permission to continue.

e. **Bathroom:** Ask if client needs to use bathroom before you start.

f. **Bodily Contact:** Once session begins, the facilitator should try to keep bodily contact with client at all times. When tuning forks are sounded around the client, the facilitator will need to break bodily contact to do this technique.

LUNG

• HAVE CLIENT LIE FACE UP

STEP 2. VALOR®.
a. <u>**Listen to the Ohm Unison x 3 (hold tuning forks to client's ears).**</u>
b. **Shoulders.** Place 3 drops of Valor on each shoulder. Hold for 5 minutes or more until a balance of energies is felt. Place your left hand on the left shoulder and your right hand on the right shoulder.
c. **Soles of Feet.** Place 6 drops of Valor on the soles of each foot. Cross your arms so your right hand holds the right foot and your left hand holds the left foot. You will have to cross your arms to accomplish this.
d. <u>**Sound the Ohm Unison to the sole of each foot at KI 1 (Gushing Spring) and at KI 3 (Great Ravine) in the depression behind the inner ankle x 3, right foot first.**</u> We begin the Raindrop journey from a firm, grounded place within. This interval deeply roots our core essence.

STEP 3. VALOR, OREGANO, THYME, EUCALYPTUS RADIATA, MELROSE, RAVEN, MYRTLE AND RAVENSARA.
a. **Foot Vita Flex.** Vita Flex on each foot along spinal reflex points, coccyx to brain, starting with right foot. Each foot should be done with 2-3 drops per foot of each of the 8 oils in the order listed x 3.
b. <u>**Sound the Ohm Octave with Low Ohm at CV4 (Origin Pass) on the abdomen four finger-widths below the umbilicus, and Ohm at CV17 (Chest Center) in the center of the chest level with the 4th rib, x 3.**</u> This interval creates a harmonic bridge and connection between the upper and lower body, further rooting our core energy.

• HAVE CLIENT ROLL OVER TO A FACE DOWN POSITION

STEP 4. DUO: OREGANO AND THYME.*
a. **Raindrop Oregano.** Holding bottle of Oregano about six inches above the client's back, drop 4-6 drops directly on the spine from sacrum to neck.
b. **3-6-12 Feathering Straight Up Spine.** Feather stroke Oregano straight up the spine with a light touch using backs of fingernails gently brushing against client's skin. Start with 3" strokes alternately with each hand x 3 the length of the spine upwards to the atlas vertebra, then 6" strokes x 3, followed by 12" strokes x 3.
c. **Thyme Raindrop.** Repeat a. & b. above for Thyme.
d. **Feathering Straight to Sides.** After both Oregano and Thyme have been applied, starting at the sacrum, feather oils away from spine straight out nd down the sides x 3, then move up half-a-hand's width and repeat until you reach the neck and skull. Repeat this sacrum to atlas x 3.
e. **Full Length Strokes.** Long feather strokes, both hands side by side, touching with back of nail tips only along both sides of the spine, sweep full length from sacrum to base of neck, fanning out and off the shoulders x 3.

LUNG

f.   **Sound the Solar 7th with the Low Ohm on GV2 (Low Back Shu) at base of sacrum and Sun fork on GV16 (Wind Mansion) on the back of the skull one inch above the posterior hairline.**
This interval assists the core Duo of Oregano and Thyme to "heat up" the cells and cleanse them for deletion of old, redundant and useless information. These two points achieve "cranial-sacral stillpoint" from which changes can occur and a new order can be achieved.

** **Important Note.*** *Some oils (particularly Oregano and Thyme) can cause heat when in contact with the skin and react with viruses, bacteria, and toxins. This is generally a good sign that the oils are seeking out and destroying harmful aliens that hibernate in the fatty tissue and lymph nodes along the spine. However, if at any time the heat becomes unpleasant for the client, apply V-6 or other vegetable oil where indicated. Relief should be immediate. Ask the client to tell you when and where this is needed throughout the Raindrop Technique session*

STEP 5.   TRIO: EUCALYPTUS RADIATA, MELROSE AND RAVEN

a.   **Raindrop the Oils on the Back in the Order Given**. Follow steps a. & b. of STEP 4 above with Eucalyptus Radiata, Melrose and Raven instead of Oregano and Thyme.

b.   **Finger Circles.** After all three oils have been applied, apply your fingers to the laminar groove along one side of the spine, slowly progressing from sacrum to atlas, using four fingers of both hands together in a clockwise motion, pulling tissues away from spine with each circle. Then walk around table and go up other side. Alternate from side to side, right to left, until both sides have been done x 3. Apply AromaSiez® where tense muscles are discovered.

c.   **Sound Zodiac 3rd wherever muscle knots are found at least x 3 at each location.**
If it is too painful to use the forks at the same location, then one fork can be placed on either side of the location of spasm.

Note on Additional Oils: *At this point, before the finger circles, additional oils (such as Joy®, Frankincense, Release®, Relieve It®, Harmony®, Panaway®, etc.) may be applied if desired according to the wishes, needs, or special circumstances of the client. With each additional oil, drop them raindrop-style directly on the spine and then stroke them straight up the spine with the 3-6-12 feathering described in STEPS 4a and 4b. described above.* **If other oils are added, sound the High Full Moon 6th near the client's ears, circle around head, then move in a figure eight over the client, from crown to feet and back to the crown x 3.** *Relax and know that the cleansing and release are perfect and enjoy a sense of magic and fulfillment, with a pull towards healing that allows one's potential to manifest.*

88

LUNG

STEP 6.   MYRTLE.

a. **Sprinkle Myrtle.** Sprinkle Myrtle oil directly on the spine with a salt-shaker-like motion from sacrum to neck.

b. **3-6-12 Feathering Straight Up Spine**. Feather straight up spine as described in STEP 4b. x 3.

c. **Thumb Vita Flex**. Thumb Vita Flex along sides of spine from sacrum to atlas x 3.

d. **Saw Maneuver & Skull-Pull.** Apply saw maneuver from sacrum to neck with three skull-pulls x 3.

e. **Spine Stretch & Shake (or Quiver)**. Apply two-handed spine stretch maneuver vibrating with a shaking or quivering motion perpendicular to the spine with each stretch, moving gradually upwards from sacrum to atlas. 3x.

f. <u>**Sound the Full Moon 6th on the Huato Jiaji points up the spine from sacrum to base of skull. The Huato Jiaji points are found on either side of the spine between the vertebrae. Then hold both forks together at GV20 (Hundred Convergences) in the depression at the crown of the head and also near the ears to allow client to hear the interval.**</u>

This interval builds yin energy, which moistens, consolidates and cools the body. It is especially effective for lung dryness that may come from smoking or emphysema.

STEP 7.   ORTHO EASE®.

a. **Apply Ortho Ease Oil**. Dispense oil generously onto palms first, then apply over the entire back, spreading it with flat palms of the hands in clockwise circular movements from hips to neck, cross over, and then back down to the hips. Repeat x 3. A free style anointing without structure or counting may be done. Include attention of the shoulder blades, neck, trapezium muscles, and places that are tight or sore. Ask client if they have any particular requests in this regard.

b. **(Optional) Rest** Quietly rest face down for 4-5 minutes. Cover with sheet to keep client warm and comfortable, if necessary. Apply more Ortho Ease as needed, repeating step 7a.

c. **Indian Rub**. Perform see-saw rub maneuver across the spine progressing from sacrum to neck and from neck to sacrum, up and down the back at least x 3. Except for step 7a. above, this is the only procedure performed both up and down the back. All others are done up only, from sacrum to neck.

d. <u>**Sound the High Jupiter 4th near the client's ears, circle around head, then move in a figure eight over the client, from crown to feet and back to the crown x 3.**</u>

The major energetic work of a Raindrop session has been done, and we relax for a few minutes to enjoy the bounty of it all.

STEP 8.   VALOR®.
a.   **Sprinkle Valor**. Sprinkle Valor oil directly on the spine with salt-shaker-like motion from sacrum to neck. Valor is a mild oil blend that does not get hot and can be applied generously.
b.   **3-6-12 Feathering Straight Up Spine**. Feather straight up spine as described STEP 4b. x 3.
c.   **Arched Feather Strokes (Angel Wings)**. Feather with backs of fingernails in a curved fanning motion arched up and out to sides in 3" strokes (3x), 6" strokes (3x) and 12" strokes (3x).
d.   **Full Length Strokes**. Long feather strokes from sacrum up to and off of the shoulders as described in STEP 4e. 3x.
e.   **Sound the High New Moon 5th near the client's ears, circle around head, then move in a figure eight over the client, from crown to feet and back to the crown x 3.**
This intervals opens, releases and dispels the stagnant energy that has accumulated during the Raindrop session, and is especially useful for asthma and lung congestion.

STEP 9.   RAVENSARA (use oil sparingly in this step, no more than 2-4 drops)
a.   **Raindrop Ravensara Oil**. Holding bottle of Ravensara about six inches above the client's back, drop only 2-3 drops directly on the spine from sacrum to neck.
b.   **3-6-12 Feathering Straight Up Spine**. Same procedure as Step 8b.
c.   **Arched Feather Strokes (Angel Wings)**. Same procedure as Step 8c.
d.   **Full Length Strokes**. Same procedure as Step 8d.

STEP 10.   HOT COMPRESS.
a.   **Dry Towel**. Place large dry bath towel covering client's back from hips to atlas.
b.   **Hot Damp Towel**. Fold smaller towel into thirds, and roll into a cylinder. Then soak with hot water from the tap, wrung nearly dry, but still enough dampness to retain heat. Unroll the hot towel over the length of the spine from neck to hips.
    * Multiple Sclerosis (MS). For people with MS, use a cold pack, NOT a hot pack. A towel soaked in cold water will do. An ice pack is also okay.
c.   **Another Dry Towel**. Lay another large towel over the compress to hold in heat.
d.   **Sound the Full Moon Major 6th near the client's ears, circle around head, then move in a figure eight over the client, from crown to feet and back to the crown x 3.**
Relax and know that the cleansing and release are perfect as the Venus energy brings the session to fullness.

LUNG

e. **Sound the Ohm Octave to the sole of each foot at KI 1 (Gushing Spring) x 3, right foot first.**

The Ohm Octave brings feelings of comfort, completeness, and creates a sense of unity with All That Is. Thus ends our journey of healing with a Raindrop Technique session.

f. **Cooking the Client**. Oils will heat up and peak out in 5-8 minutes. If heat becomes too uncomfortable, apply V-6 or vegetable oil where needed. (See Note in Step 4.) Ask client to tell you when oils have cooled to a comfortable level.

g. **If Not Hot Enough**. If oils do not heat up with client, facilitator may place hands on back over the towel. NOTE: Because ravensara oil has been applied last, the client may experience what feels like coolness when, in fact, their back is warm.

STEP 11. REST & WATER

a. **Rest Quietly**. At this point client may wish to relax quietly for a few minutes. Whenever ready, they may sit up slowly with the facilitator standing nearby, being careful as they get off the massage table assisted by the facilitator.

b. **Drinking Water.** Have the client immediately drink a glass or bottle of good water and urge them to drink plenty of water for the next week.

STEP 12. RE-EVALUATION AND RE-MEASUREMENT.

a. **Measure Height Afterwards**. Re-measure client's height barefooted. Most will have grown from 1/4 to 1/2 inch. Those with severe spinal curvature may grow an inch or more. The benefits of Raindrop may not always include immediate growth but can be experienced by the receiver in other ways.

b. **Adjustments Continue for a Week.** A complete evaluation of the benefits received from Raindrop Technique may take several days to assess.

c. **Drink Lots of Water.** Remind the client to drink lots of water. The recommended amount is to divide their weight in pounds by two and drink that amount in ounces of pure (non-chlorinated) water every day.

---

* These notes correspond to a 120-min DVD entitled *Raindrop Technique*.
Available from CARE, RR 4 Box 646, Marble Hill, MO 63764
• (800) 758-8629 • or visit www.RaindropTraining.com.
Price: $29.95 + $9 s&h • Includes a set of notes

91

Additional Essential Oils
Used in Raindrop Technique for Longevity

All of the Systems-specific Raindrop Technique protocol use Valor, oregano and thyme as the core three oils to open and close Raindrop Technique (EDOR, 4th Ed, page 299). Basil, marjoram, wintergreen, cypress and peppermint are replaced with oils more specific to the body system being treated. Details about the specific oils used to focus on the **Longevity** system are included below.

ORANGE (*Citrus sinensis*)--Family: Rutaceae (citrus); boosts immunity, used for arteriosclerosis, hypertension, cancer and fluid retention. Contains over 90% limonene, which has been studied for its ability to combat tumor growth in over 50 clinical studies.

Orange is cooling with an affinity for Lung, Heart and Stomach meridians. Use it to Release Wind Heat with fever, chills, and cough; Clear Heart Fire with palpitations, hypertension and insomnia; and to Descend Stomach qi to promote peristalsis and clear symptoms of Stomach Fire (indigestion, nausea, IBS).

CLOVE (*Syzygium aromaticum*)--Family: myrtle family; anti-aging, cardiovascular disease, anticoagulant properties. Contains 70-85% phenols which cleanse cellular receptor sites.

Hot by nature, Clove has an affinity for the Spleen, Stomach and Kidney meridians. It can be used to warm the Kidneys to treat bone, teeth and impotence; warm the interior to expel Cold in the Stomach and Spleen to treat digestive problems and abdominal pain. Clove also improves thyroid and immune function by strengthening Deficient Spleen and Kidney qi.

LONGEVITY® (contains clove, thyme, orange, and frankincense); has the highest antioxidant and DNA-protecting essential oils, promotes longevity and prevents premature aging. Clove has the highest known antioxidant power as measured by ORAC (oxygen radical absorbent capacity), a test developed by USDA researchers at Tufts University. Thyme has been shown to dramatically boost glutathione levels in the heart, liver, and brain. The oxidation of fats in the body is directly linked to accelerated aging, and thyme prevents peroxidation of fats found in many vital organs.

FRANKINCENSE (*Boswellia carteri*)--Family: Burseraceae (frankincense); anti-tumoral, immunostimulant, antidepressant; increases spiritual awareness, promotes meditation, improves attitude. Contains 64-90% monoterpenes, 5-10% sesquiterpenes, which stimulate the limbic system of the brain (the center of memory and emotions), and the hypothalamus, pineal and pituitary glands.

Slightly cooling and drying, Frankincense has an affinity for the Lung, Heart and Kidney meridians. Use it for Lung Heat with Chest Qi Stasis symptoms of agitation, anxiety and irritability. Clears heat in the Lungs with coughing or wheezing, Stomach with ulcers, and Kidneys with cystitis. It can also reduce swelling and treat non-healing wounds, ulcers and scars.

PEPPERMINT (*Mentha piperita*) CT menthol - Family: Lamiaceae supports digestive system, respiratory system, and nervous system. Has been used for headaches. Research has shown that inhaling peppermint improves concentration and mental retention. Detoxifying to the liver. A synergistic oil that supports and improves the beneficial actions of other oils used in conjunction. High in phenolics, but contains 9% sesquiterpenes.

Peppermint has an affinity for the Lung and Liver meridians with its cooling energy. Clears Wind Heat of headaches, fever, sore throat, and dry cough, as well as regulates Liver qi to promote menstruation, and decongest the Liver/PMS. It also promotes the movement of Wei qi.

Additional Intervals
Used in Longevity Raindrop Technique

Fifth, 2:3
Earth Day/Ohm - highly energetic, full of movement, intense propelling energy, joyful. Also considered to be an Augmented 4th or Diminished 5th. This interval has also been called Crux Ansata, a transition point where spirit is redeemed from matter. This interval is the most fundamental for building energy and eliminating fatigue. If there is a particular Energy Center (nerve plexus/chakra) that is weak, sound the forks extra times at that level of the spine.
High Neptune/High Ohm - a near Perfect Fifth, aptly called the Ecstatic Fifth, opens and moves the visionary from transpersonal to transcendental, fulfills the yearning for connection with the Infinite. Because of Neptune's association with the spinal canal and spinal cord, we bring the Raindrop session nearly to completion with this interval in sweeping motions the length of the spine and to the feet.

LONGEVITY
Vibrational Raindrop

Based on Raindrop Technique as Taught by D. Gary Young
At the Young Living Level I Training Conference in
Dallas, Texas, January 25-29, 2000
(From the CARE Raindrop Training Notes)

**The notes in Underlined Helvetica Bold are the tuning fork applications
to be done with the Longevity Raindrop Tuning Kit**

• **NOTE:**   The person receiving oils is called the "client" or the "receiver." The person administering the oils is called the "facilitator." While this is the version of Raindrop taught by CARE Instructors, you may adapt the tuning forks to be used after the appropriate oils in different versions of Raindrop.

• **PRELIMINARIES:** Facilitator should trim nails as short as possible and file sharp corners and edges. Facilitator and client should both remove all metal, especially rings, bracelets, and watches.

STEP 1.   EVALUATION, PREPARATION AND PERMISSION.

a.   **Measure Height** of the client barefooted using a square box against a wall and sliding down to the head to assure a level measurement. This is not an essential part of raindrop, but is an objective demonstration of what often happens. Most people grow a little with a raindrop, but if one does not grow, that does not mean the raindrop has been ineffective or erroneously per formed.

b.   **Allergies, Sensitivities, Toxicity, etc.** Ask if client is prone to allergies, reactions to drugs or has developed any sensitizations to any sub stances. Mention to the client that allergic reactions to therapeutic grade essential oils are not possible, but sometimes there can be a detox reaction. Ask if they smoke or if they have ever engaged in occu pations exposing them to chemicals such as beauty shop, auto body, professional housecleaning, pesticides, herbicides, photo chemicals, environmental engineering, hospitals, etc.

c.   **Suggested Resources with Cleansing Information**: *Essential Oils Desk Reference*; *Reference Guide for Essential Oils*; *Healing for the Age of Enlightenment*.

d.   **Ask Permission.** After explaining the procedure to the client, ask per mission to continue.

e.   **Bathroom:** Ask if client needs to use bathroom before you start.

f.   **Bodily Contact:** Once session begins, the facilitator should try to keep bodily contact with client at all times. When tuning forks are sound ed around the client, the facilitator will need to break bodily contact to do this technique.

LONGEVITY

• **HAVE CLIENT LIE FACE UP**

STEP 2.   VALOR®.

a.   **Listen to the Ohm Unison x 3 (hold tuning forks to client's ears).**

b.   **Shoulders.** Place 3 drops of Valor on each shoulder. Hold for 5 minutes or more until a balance of energies is felt. Place your left hand on the left shoulder and your right hand on the right shoulder.

c.   **Soles of Feet.** Place 6 drops of Valor on the soles of each foot. Cross your arms so your right hand holds the right foot and your left hand holds the left foot. You will have to cross your arms to accomplish this.

d.   **Sound the Ohm Unison to the sole of each foot at KI 1 (Gushing Spring) and at KI 3 (Great Ravine) in the depression behind the inner ankle x 3, right foot first.** We begin the Raindrop journey from a firm, grounded place within. This interval deeply roots our core essence.

STEP 3.   VALOR, OREGANO, THYME, ORANGE, CLOVE, LONGEVITY, FRANKINCENSE and PEPPERMINT.

a.   **Foot Vita Flex.** Vita Flex on each foot along spinal reflex points, coccyx to brain, starting with right foot. Each foot should be done with 2-3 drops per foot of each of the 8 oils in the order listed x 3.

b.   **Sound the Ohm Octave with Low Ohm at CV4 (Origin Pass) on the abdomen four finger-widths below the umbilicus, and Ohm at CV17 (Chest Center) in the center of the chest level with the 4th rib, x 3.**
      This interval creates a harmonic bridge and connection between the upper and lower body, further rooting our core energy.

• **HAVE CLIENT ROLL OVER TO A FACE DOWN POSITION**

STEP 4.   DUO: OREGANO AND THYME.*

a.   **Raindrop Oregano**. Holding bottle of Oregano about six inches above the client's back, drop 4-6 drops directly on the spine from sacrum to neck.

b.   **3-6-12 Feathering Straight Up Spine.** Feather stroke Oregano straight up the spine with a light touch using backs of fingernails gently brushing against client's skin. Start with 3" strokes alternately with each hand x 3 the length of the spine upwards to the atlas vertebra, then 6" strokes x 3, followed by 12" strokes x 3.

c.   **Thyme Raindrop.** Repeat a. & b. above for Thyme.

d.   **Feathering Straight to Sides.** After both Oregano and Thyme have been applied, starting at the sacrum, feather oils away from spine straight out nd down the sides x 3, then move up half-a-hand's width and repeat until you reach the neck and skull. Repeat this sacrum to atlas x 3.

e.   **Full Length Strokes.** Long feather strokes, both hands side by side, touching with back of nail tips only along both sides of the spine, sweep full length from sacrum to base of neck, fanning out and off the shoulders x 3.

f. **Sound the Solar 7th with the Low Ohm on GV2 (Low Back Shu) at base of sacrum and Sun fork on GV16 (Wind Mansion) on the back of the skull one inch above the posterior hairline.**
This interval assists the core Duo of Oregano and Thyme to "heat up" the cells and cleanse them for deletion of old, redundant and useless information. These two points achieve "cranial-sacral stillpoint" from which changes can occur and a new order can be achieved.

* Important Note. Some oils (particularly Oregano and Thyme) can cause heat when in contact with the skin and react with viruses, bacteria, and toxins. This is generally a good sign that the oils are seeking out and destroying harmful aliens that hibernate in the fatty tissue and lymph nodes along the spine. However, if at any time the heat becomes unpleasant for the client, apply V-6 or other vegetable oil where indicated. Relief should be immediate. Ask the client to tell you when and where this is needed throughout the Raindrop Technique session

STEP 5.   TRIO: ORANGE, CLOVE, AND LONGEVITY
a. **Raindrop the Oils on the Back in the Order Given**. Follow steps
a. & b. of STEP 4 above with Orange, Clove and Longevity instead
of Oregano and Thyme.
b. **Finger Circles**. After all three oils have been applied, apply your fingers to the laminar groove along one side of the spine, slowly progressing from sacrum to atlas, using four fingers of both hands together in a clockwise motion, pulling tissues away from spine with each circle. Then walk around table and go up other side. Alternate from side to side, right to left, until both sides have been done x 3. Apply AromaSiez® where tense muscles are discovered.
c. **Sound Zodiac 3rd wherever muscle knots are found at least x 3 at each location.**
If it is too painful to use the forks at the same location, then one fork can be placed on either side of the location of spasm.

Note on Additional Oils: *At this point, before the finger circles, additional oils (such as Joy®, Frankincense, Release®, Relieve It®, Harmony®, Panaway®, etc.) may be applied if desired according to the wishes, needs, or special circumstances of the client. With each additional oil, drop them raindrop-style directly on the spine and then stroke them straight up the spine with the 3-6-12 feathering described in STEPS 4a and 4b. described above. **If other oils are added, sound the High Full Moon 6th near the client's ears, circle around head, then move in a figure eight over the client, from crown to feet and back to the crown x 3.** Relax and know that the cleansing and release are perfect and enjoy a sense of magic and fulfillment, with a pull towards healing that allows one's potential to manifest.*

STEP 6.   FRANKINCENSE.

a.   **Sprinkle Frankincense.** Sprinkle Frankincense oil directly on the spine with a salt-shaker-like motion from sacrum to neck.

b.   **3-6-12 Feathering Straight Up Spine.** Feather straight up spine as described in STEP 4b. x 3.

c.   **Thumb Vita Flex**. Thumb Vita Flex along sides of spine from sacrum to atlas x 3.

d.   **Saw Maneuver & Skull-Pull**. Apply saw maneuver from sacrum to neck with three skull-pulls x 3.

e.   **Spine Stretch & Shake (or Quiver).** Apply two-handed spine stretch maneuver vibrating with a shaking or quivering motion perpendicular to the spine with each stretch, moving gradually upwards from sacrum to atlas. 3x.

f.   **Sound the Earth Day 5th on the Huato Jiaji points up the spine from sacrum to base of skull. The Huato Jiaji points are found on either side of the spine between the vertebrae. Then hold both forks together at GV20 (Hundred Convergences) in the depression at the crown of the head and also near the ears to allow client to hear the interval.**
This interval is the most fundamental for building energy and eliminating fatigue. If there is a particular Energy Center (nerve plexus/chakra) that s weak, sound the forks extra times at that level of the spine.

STEP 7.   ORTHO EASE®.

a.   **Apply Ortho Ease Oil.** Dispense oil generously onto palms first, then apply over the entire back, spreading it with flat palms of the hands in clockwise circular movements from hips to neck, cross over, and then back down to the hips. Repeat x 3. A free style anointing without structure or counting may be done. Include attention of the shoulder blades, neck, trapezium muscles, and places that are tight or sore. Ask client if they have any particular requests in this regard.

b.   **(Optional) Rest** Quietly rest face down for 4-5 minutes. Cover with sheet to keep client warm and comfortable, if necessary. Apply more Ortho Ease as needed, repeating step 7a.

c.   **Indian Rub.** Perform see-saw rub maneuver across the spine progressing from sacrum to neck and from neck to sacrum, up and down the back at least x 3. Except for step 7a. above, this is the only procedure performed both up and down the back. All others are done up only, from sacrum to neck.

d.   **Sound the High Jupiter 4th near the client's ears, circle around head, then move in a figure eight over the client, from crown to feet and back to the crown x 3.**
The major energetic work of a Raindrop session has been done, and we relax for a few minutes to enjoy the bounty of it all.

LONGEVITY

STEP 8.   VALOR®.

a.   Sprinkle Valor. Sprinkle Valor oil directly on the spine with salt-shaker-like motion from sacrum to neck. Valor is a mild oil blend that does not get hot and can be applied generously.

b.   3-6-12 Feathering Straight Up Spine. Feather straight up spine as described STEP 4b. x 3.

c.   Arched Feather Strokes (Angel Wings). Feather with backs of fingernails in a curved fanning motion arched up and out to sides in 3" strokes (3x), 6" strokes (3x) and 12" strokes (3x).

d.   Full Length Strokes. Long feather strokes from sacrum up to and off of the shoulders as described in STEP 4e. 3x.

e.   <u>Sound the High Neptune 5th near the client's ears, circle around head, then move in a figure eight over the client, from crown to feet and back to the crown x 3.</u>
Because of Neptune's association with the spinal canal and spinal cord, we bring the Raindrop session nearly to completion with this interval in sweeping motions the length of the spine and to the feet.

STEP 9.   PEPPERMINT (use oil sparingly in this step, no more than 2-4 drops)

a.   Raindrop Peppermint Oil. Holding bottle of Peppermint about six inches above the client's back, drop only 2-3 drops directly on the spine from sacrum to neck.

b.   3-6-12 Feathering Straight Up Spine. Same procedure as Step 8b.

c.   Arched Feather Strokes (Angel Wings). Same procedure as Step 8c.

d.   Full Length Strokes. Same procedure as Step 8d.

STEP 10.   HOT COMPRESS.

a.   Dry Towel. Place large dry bath towel covering client's back from hips to atlas.

b.   Hot Damp Towel. Fold smaller towel into thirds, and roll into a cylinder. Then soak with hot water from the tap, wrung nearly dry, but still enough dampness to retain heat. Unroll the hot towel over the length of the spine from neck to hips.
* Multiple Sclerosis (MS). For people with MS, use a cold pack, NOT a hot pack. A towel soaked in cold water will do. An ice pack is also okay.

c.   Another Dry Towel. Lay another large towel over the compress to hold in heat.

d.   <u>Sound the Full Moon Major 6th near the client's ears, circle around head, then move in a figure eight over the client, from crown to feet and back to the crown x 3.</u>
Relax and know that the cleansing and release are perfect as the Venus energy brings the session to fullness.

e.   **Sound the Ohm Octave to the sole of each foot at KI 1 (Gushing Spring) x 3, right foot first.**
     The Ohm Octave brings feelings of comfort, completeness, and creates a sense of unity with All That Is. Thus ends our journey of healing with a Raindrop Technique session.

f.   **Cooking the Client**. Oils will heat up and peak out in 5-8 minutes. If heat becomes too uncomfortable, apply V-6 or vegetable oil where needed. (See Note in Step 4.) Ask client to tell you when oils have cooled to a comfortable level.

g.   **If Not Hot Enough**. If oils do not heat up with client, facilitator may place hands on back over the towel. NOTE: Because peppermint oil has been applied last, the client may experience what feels like coolness when, in fact, their back is warm.

STEP 11.   REST & WATER

a.   **Rest Quietly**. At this point client may wish to relax quietly for a few minutes. Whenever ready, they may sit up slowly with the facilitator standing nearby, being careful as they get off the massage table assisted by the facilitator.

b.   **Drinking Water.** Have the client immediately drink a glass or bottle of good water and urge them to drink plenty of water for the next week.

STEP 12.   RE-EVALUATION AND RE-MEASUREMENT.

a.   **Measure Height Afterwards**. Re-measure client's height barefooted. Most will have grown from 1/4 to 1/2 inch. Those with severe spinal curvature may grow an inch or more. The benefits of Raindrop may not always include immediate growth but can be experienced by the receiver in other ways.

b.   **Adjustments Continue for a Week.** A complete evaluation of the benefits received from Raindrop Technique may take several days to assess.

c.   **Drink Lots of Water.** Remind the client to drink lots of water. The recommended amount is to divide their weight in pounds by two and drink that amount in ounces of pure (non-chlorinated) water every day.

---

* These notes correspond to a 120-min DVD entitled *Raindrop Technique.*
Available from CARE, RR 4 Box 646, Marble Hill, MO 63764
• (800) 758-8629 • or visit www.RaindropTraining.com.
Price: $29.95 + $9 s&h • Includes a set of notes

Selected Bibliography

Beaulieu, John, *Human Tuning*, New York, NY: Biosonic Enterprises, 2010

Beaulieu, John, *Music and Sound in the Healing Arts*, Barrytown, NY: Station Hill Press, 1987

Berendt, Joachim-Ernstt, *The World is Sound*, Nada Brahma, Rochester, VT: Destiny Books, 1883

Burroughs, Stanley, *Healing for the Age of Enlightenment*, Newcastle, CA: 1976

Carey, Donna, and de Muynk, Marjorie, *Acutonics: There's no place like Ohm*, Vadito, NM: Devachan Press, 2002

Carey, Donna, et.al., *Acutonics: From Galaxies to Cells*, Llano, NM: Devachan Press, 2010

Cousto, Hans, *The Cosmic Octave: Origin of Harmony*, Mendocino, CA: LifeRhythm, 2000

Elliott, S; Minsum, K; Beaulieu, J; Stefano, G, "*Sound therapy induced relaxation: down regulating stress processes and pathologies*", Med Sci Monit, 2003; 9(5): RA116-121, as reprinted in Human Tuning

Emoto, Masaru, *The Hidden Messages in Water*, Hillsboro, OR: Beyond Words Publishing, 2004.

Goldman, Jonathan, *Shifting Frequencies*, Flagstaff, AZ: Light Technology Publishing, 1998

Goldman, Jonathan, *Healing Sounds: The Power of Harmonics*, Rochester, VT: Healing Arts Press, 1992

Hesse, Hermann, *Magister Ludi*, New York, NY: Bantam, 1982

Higley, Alan and Connie, *Reference Guide to Essential Oils*, Twelfth Edition, Spanish Fork, UT: Abundant Health, 2010

Jenny, Hans, *Cymatics*, Newmarket, NH: MACROmedia, 2001

Lauterwasser, Alexander, *Water Sound Images*, Newmarket, NH: MACROmedia 2002

Manwaring, Brian, Ed., *Essential Oils Desk Reference*, 4th Edition, 2009

Prigogine, Ilya, *Order Out of Chaos*, New York, NY: Bantam Books, 1984

Stewart, David, *A Statistical Validation of Raindrop Technique*, Marble Hill, MO: Care Publications, 2003

Stewart, David, *The Chemistry of Essential Oils Made Simple*, Marble Hill, MO: Care Publications, 2005 and 2006

Young, D. Gary, *Essential Oils Integrative Medical Guide*, Essential Science Publishing, 2006

Young, D. Gary, *Raindrop Technique*, Essential Science Publishing, 2008

Resources

Tuning Forks

For more information about the tuning forks used in this book, please visit www.AromaSounds.com

Essential Oils

For more information about Young Living Essential Oils, please visit www.AromaSounds.com

Classes

More than 150 CARE classes are taught each year all over the world. They include classes on Oils of Scripture, Applied Vitaflex, Raindrop Technique, Chemistry of Essential Oils, and Emotional Releasing with Oils. An up-to-date list of Certified CARE Instructors, as well as a calendar of seminars, can be found on the website, www.RaindropTraining.com.

Books

A Statistical Validation of Raindrop Technique,
Available from CARE, RR 4 Box 646, Marble Hill, MO 63764 • (800) 758-8629 • or visit www.RaindropTraining.com. $9.95 + $5 s&h

The Chemistry of Essential Oils Made Simple,
Available from CARE, RR 4 Box 646, Marble Hill, MO 63764 • (800) 758-8629 • or visit www.RaindropTraining.com. $49.95 + $9 s&h

DVDs

Applied Vitaflex, Available from CARE, RR 4 Box 646, Marble Hill, MO 63764 • (800) 758-8629 • or visit www.RaindropTraining.com. $29.95 + $9 s&h

Raindrop Technique, Available from CARE, RR 4 Box 646, Marble Hill, MO 63764 • (800) 758-8629 • or visit www.RaindropTraining.com. $29.95 + $9 s&h

CDs

Jonathan Goldman at www.HealingSounds.com
Andrew Weil and Kimba Arem at www.SoundsTrue.com

Art

Charles Wildbank at www.wildbank.com

About the Author

Christi Bonds-Garrett, M.A., M.D. has been offering Integrative Medical care since 1995, and has treated over 6000 patients from this perspective. She received both her Master's Degree in Counseling and Medical Degree from the University of Nevada in Reno. After completing an Internship in Psychiatry in West Virginia, she completed a Residency in Family Practice in 1992, as well as becoming Board Certified in Family Medicine in 1993. For over 15 years she has specialized in Women's Health Care, utilizing unique combinations of herbs, oils, tuning forks/singing bowls, and western medications to help bring her female patients to a better internal balance.

While working as Medical Director for three Native American Clinics near Yosemite, California in the 1990s, she pursued advanced studies in Chinese Herbs, Nutrition, Medical Acupuncture at UCLA, and Homeopathy at the National Center of Homeopathy in Washington DC. Dr. Bonds-Garrett was a licensed Homeopathic Physician in the state of Nevada and testified to the Nevada State Board of Medical Examiners on behalf of the merits of Integrative Medicine.

More recently, she completed a two-year Fellowship in Integrative Medicine through the University of Arizona under the direction of Dr. Andrew Weil. Her special interests include tapping the healing potential within through the use of creative activities.

She is a Certified CARE Instructor and teaches classes on Raindrop Technique and the therapeutic use of essential oils. Dr. Bonds-Garrett is currently writing several more books on the application of vibrational medicine and essential oils, applied to esoteric styles of acupuncture. She has a private practice in the Lowertown Arts District of the historic town of Paducah, Kentucky.